Strength Training Over 40

A Practical Guide to Building and Maintaining a
Healthier, Leaner, and Stronger Body

Baz Thompson

Table of Contents

Introduction

If you are over the age of 40 and are committed to getting into shape whether it's for the first time or you want to return to the physical condition of when you were younger, you have taken an important first step: the objective of this book is to help you attain a stronger, leaner body leading to better health and well-being, and to get you there safely and effectively with exercise routines and lifestyle improvements you can easily adopt and follow.

You are right to want to build a strong, lean body, exchanging fat for muscle mass, building strength and endurance, improving your health, and increasing your disease resistance. People over 40 can become strong and fit, but the exercise routines to get them there are not the same as when they were 20 or 25, Your body has changed, yet with the correct, scientifically evolved, and tested training techniques, you will be surprised how soon you will see and feel real progress.

You'll be impressed to know how many people over 40 who were not satisfied with their bodies and physical conditions have decided they would commit to shape up, do it right, and get the results they want. Their positive results include building lean muscle mass, getting more definition, reducing fat, especially around the belly, increasing energy and endurance, and feeling better about themselves. It can work for you as your state of mind will improve with a greater feeling of self-esteem, reduced anxiety, and a positive belief that anything is possible no matter your age.

What Are Your Fitness Goals?

Do you want to be proud when you look in a mirror and see muscles returning after being soft and hidden under a layer of flab? Or see that your potbelly has diminished as your abs become more defined? Are you among the two-thirds of Americans who are overweight or obese, and you want to lose the excess weight as an investment in your overall health and longevity?

Now that you are over 40, do you realize that has your cardiovascular health should be a priority? Do you know that heart disease becomes a risk as middle-age progresses? That heart attacks and strokes can be averted with the proper conditioning and dietary practices?

It's Up to You: Motivation and Commitment

Achievement of your muscle- and strength-building goals and attainment of real physical fitness are dependent upon the levels of your motivation and commitment. It's important to understand that you'll be exercising at least several days per week with resistance training that may involve lifting, pulling, and stretching, plus raising your heart rate for sustained periods through cardio, or aerobic, exercises. Be assured that with the training advice you receive here, these routines will not take up much time and are easy to learn with our instructions.

Ask yourself why you want to get into shape and achieve your physical fitness goals. What is motivating you? There is no right or wrong reason for your commitment. What matters is that you have the drive and tenacity to stay with it, starting from the initial first exercises, then gradually increasing to more intensive routines. You will not be alone as you join the many others who have recognized the value of middle-age strength training.

Resistance exercises can be performed in fitness centers or your home. You can do body calisthenics in a small easy-to-assemble home gym. You also can do them without dumbbells, barbells, cables, and machines. What matters most is not the equipment, but rather your commitment to follow the instructions and perform the exercises. Don't let yourself become one of those people who joins a fitness center, buys equipment, but never follows through. Good intentions are one thing; motivation and commitment are another.

This Book is Your Roadmap

This book will enable you to achieve your fitness goals. It recognizes the need to present the most effective exercise routines for you while respecting your age and current fitness level. Whether you are just turning age 40, or are well beyond, the benefits of resistance and cardiovascular conditioning are clinically proven to be beneficial at every age. Also, as you mature, good dietary practices take on added importance to your health and longevity

The motivations that ignite your desire to begin a strengthening and conditioning program need to be strong enough to keep you committed to turn physical fitness and muscle-building into an integral lifestyle component. That is why we are providing step-by-step training, options to fit your personal preferences, and the availability of where and how to train.

You Have the Time

Too often we hear the excuse, "I don't have time to work out," and this may be expressed by men and women at any age. The reality is they either are not motivated to get into a workout routine or deeply committed to keeping it going and making it part of their lifestyle. They have not accepted how essential their strength and fitness workouts are for their health and wellness, for how they look, and for how they feel. It takes inner psychological strength to face those weights and cables, treadmill or exercise bike at daybreak or before lunch or dinner.

No one ever ends a good workout session feeling it was a waste of time. On the contrary, they're pumped up by the satisfaction of lifting weights correctly, getting their heart rate up, and their arteries flowing along with the "high" that comes from the beta-endorphin hormones that vigorous exercise releases.

Exercises Targeted to Your Age

This book was written for you at a stage in your life when your physical condition and overall shape are not what they used to be. The exercises to build muscles, and get you into great shape, are not the same as those you did when you were younger. We've done the research to identify the types of exercises and routines that are best for you now. You will learn how to get started, which exercises are best to get you started, how often to train, when to rest and recover, and how to progress. You will learn the fundamental exercises for optimal results while avoiding complicated, potentially harmful exercises best left for professionals.

All strengthening exercises in this book are explained and demonstrated, so you will have no difficulties in learning how to perform the movements correctly.

As we age, our exercise needs evolve, too. Certain muscle groups need more attention to keep our guts flat, to help protect our backs from soreness and pain, to help us improve our balance, and to help prevent falls that can cause hip fractures and other serious injuries. Middle-age weightlifting may require a more careful selection of weights, movements, repetitions, and rest periods between sets. As you will see, the core of muscle building is hypertrophy, which is the breaking down of muscle fibers, and the subsequent repair and rebuilding. Rest is essential for this process to succeed. Our training plans consider all these factors so you don't have to worry about them.

Overview by Chapters

This book is organized to guide you through the nature of your body now that you have reached middle-age. It will show you that while your body is different than it was, you are still able to lift weights, use muscle-building equipment, and perform bodyweight calisthenics to build lean, well-defined muscle mass and grow stronger. You will be guided through cardiovascular exercises you can perform to get into great physical condition. Your diet will play an important role in your health and muscle-building, and the overriding principles are the motivation to start and the commitment to stay with it.

Chapter 1 will help you gain an appreciation of how your body has evolved and how at age 40 or older, it is not the same as it was at 20 or 25. Unless, of course, you've been working out continuously with progressively heavier weights, which most of us certainly have not been doing. The majority of us has become more sedentary: riding instead of walking and running, sitting instead of standing, and no longer lifting the weights and doing the calisthenics that kept our muscles firm and our bodies lean. Our bodies have followed our lead and slowed, leaving us with less lean muscle mass and more body fat, showing itself in a growing waistline. This adds up to you not being able to pick up where you left off and lift weights and do intense exercises like you used to.

Chapter 2 will convince you that your age is not a barrier to achieving ambitious muscle-building goals. It's well established that you can build lean, strong muscles at age 40 and beyond. It's just a matter of performing the right exercises with the right weights and routines. Muscle and strength-building is a matter of applying scientific and effective principles that reduce the risk of injury while optimizing results in the shortest time. It is definitely not too late to get started, and now is an excellent time to make the commitment and start lifting.

Chapter 3 will reassure you of your ability to lift heavy weights despite what you might have heard. Being a middle-aged weightlifter does not mean you cannot lift heavy weights, or that heavier weights are for youngsters and you need to lighten up. Opinions are one thing, and experience and research are another. The evidence, based on extensive training and coaching, is that heavy weights are the way to go at middle-age. You will meet action-hero celebrities whom you admire and who will share workouts with you that helped propel them to superstar status. You will see that if your goal is to build lean, well-defined muscle mass, heavy weights are the right weights as long as they aren't too heavy.

Chapter 4 covers your exercise selection and recovery routine. You will be doing exercises with heavy weights, but they will not necessarily be the same exercises you performed when you were younger or that you see someone else doing at the fitness center. Some weightlifting exercises are safe for you at this age. Others that you may have once performed are now too risky and need to be avoided. Recovery time after hard exertion was important when you were younger to enable the hypertrophy rebuilding process to function, but now it's doubly important because, after age 40, hypertrophy takes longer and the risk of injury from overwork is greater. Your patience will be rewarded with results.

Chapter 5 is about commitment. With your metabolism gradually slowing down, the need for your commitment to physical fitness and building lean muscle intensifies. With age, you lose lean muscle mass at an increased rate each year. At the same time, your body increases its storage of excess energy as fat. Your gut shows that result as you wonder, "Where did my six-pack abs go?" This is when you need to look in the mirror and make the personal commitment to go the distance. Decide there will be no excuses to keep you from becoming a muscular, strong, physically impressive person who faces middle-age with confidence.

Chapter 6 is about the importance of a healthy diet. Your health, strength, and endurance depend on the fuel you ingest, the quality and types of foods you eat. As crucial as weightlifting is to build muscles and become stronger and more fit, your diet is even more influential. The carbohydrates, proteins, and fats in your diet need to be well-sourced from healthy, more natural, less processed food that provides the essential vitamins, minerals, and antioxidants that your body needs. There is a range of diets that you can consider, but we'll introduce you to one that is more than just a diet. It's a complete lifestyle overhaul with a wide range of delicious foods that you will love without having to count calories. In recognizing that our diet plays a key role in building muscle and keeping off fat, we'll help you cut through all the dietary misinformation and embrace a lifelong dietary practice rather than a fad diet that will come and go. There are fundamentals of nutrition that you will learn to follow.

Chapter 7 will address and debunk the misconceptions that can interfere with your commitment and motivation. You'll discover that your workouts can take less time than you think. That you can put real effort and intensity into your exercise routines and get more out of your investment in time and energy. You will get a new perspective on running, walking, and other proven forms of cardiovascular conditioning, and you'll understand how diet and exercise can work synergistically to get your weight where it belongs, to help strengthen your immune system, and to prevent diseases.

About the Author

CJD Fitness founder Baz Thompson is a CYQ Master Personal Trainer who has helped hundreds of people like you achieve their fitness goals. Baz works with professional athletes in world-renowned fitness facilities as well as coaching global executives and almost everyone in between, including people of all ages who fly in from around the world to benefit from his personal training. His certifications include Kettlebell Concepts, PROnatal Fitness Pre- and Post-Natal, and TRX Level 2.

Baz realizes that too many people approach middle-age with a sense of frustration about lifting weights, building muscle, and getting back into shape. But, Baz says it doesn't have to be that way: it's not too late to get started in a well-planned weightlifting and conditioning program. If you have the motivation to take charge of your physical fitness and get into shape, to build lean muscle mass and get rid of fat, to revitalize your cardiovascular conditioning and boost your self-esteem, and feel absolutely great about yourself and how you look, this is the one roadmap that you need. This professional, step-by-step coaching on exercise and diet will help you achieve all of your fitness goals after age 40 and well beyond.

"I am excited to be your trainer, coach, and advisor on this journey to achieving strong, lean muscles that are well defined and functional as well as helping you lower your body fat level and bring your weight into a healthy range. You will be joining the hundreds of people I have trained and helped achieve their fitness and strength goals at a time in their lives when they thought it was too late for them. It was not too late for them, and it is not too late for you" – Baz Thompson (2020).

Are you ready? Let's get your fitness education and training started!

Chapter 1:

Your Body Has Evolved

A recently published online article in *WebMD* (2020) underscores the importance of exercise during middle-age and makes the point that while you no longer have the body of a 20-year-old, exercise that makes you stronger and gets you into shape is more important now than when you were younger. Being stronger and more physically fit is essential to maintaining a good quality of life and keeping your independence as you mature.

The benefits of weight training and other forms of resistance exercises, along with keeping up aerobically through cardiovascular training, are considerable for those of us who are over 40, 50, or more.

- ➤ Muscles burn more calories compared to body fat even when you are at rest. This can offset the effects of middle-age slowing of your metabolism and make it easier to keep extra pounds from adding up.

- ➤ Consistent exercise is credited with helping to slow or prevent the onset of life-threatening diseases that may begin in middle-age, including hypertension, strokes, atherosclerosis and other types of heart disease, diabetes, osteoporosis, and certain types of cancer.

- ➤ Strength and fitness training are believed to slow the progression of Alzheimer's disease and other forms of dementia as well as the cognitive decline that slows down the brain's usual sharpness.

These are the concerns that we'll address in this chapter and will guide you in how to know yourself, build up yourself, and protect yourself.

Know Thyself

The ancient Greek aphorism, "Know thyself," is engraved as a maxim on the Temple of Apollo in Delphi, and it is an appropriate prequel for your strength training over age 40. As you ramp up your motivation and commitment, it is important to pause for a moment and take stock of who you are at this point in your life.

Your body is no longer that of a teenager or young adult because with the years come physical changes. Some are due to inevitable wear and tear from life's stresses while others are results of the aging process. Your muscles are gradually atrophying, ligaments, joints, and tendons are not as flexible, and your resilience is slower, meaning it takes you longer to recover after hard exertion. Your body shape may have changed, and your midsection may be getting larger.

Other, more subtle changes may be quietly working behind the scenes and slowing down your metabolism, which is the overall rate of your body's functioning.

All of this adds up to you not being able to pick up where you left off and lift weights and do intense exercise like you used to. But it is certainly not too late to return to a full exercise and fitness program focusing on weightlifting.

You can slow the aging process through exercise and diet, rebuild lost muscle mass, build new, larger muscles, and gain appreciable strength. That's what this book is all about: restoring your body to earlier strength, building new muscle mass, increasing flexibility, getting your weight down, and keeping your arteries clear to slow the onset of cardiovascular disease.

Benchmarking 1: Measuring Up

Assessing your current condition is the best way to objectively determine where you are physically right now before beginning your weight training and overall physical improvement program. The first stage of this benchmarking assessment is how you look and measure up.

The mirror, the scale, and the tape measure are impartial judges of how well you are doing and can help you set goals for where you want to go. Begin by looking in the mirror while in your underwear and objectively consider how you look. Don't be hard on yourself; just take an assessment of where you are now and consider it a benchmark, a starting point. Check out your upper arms: how firm and defined are the biceps upfront, and the triceps behind? Are your chest muscles, the pectorals or "pecs," starting to sag? Next, is there any definition to your abdominal muscles or sign of the famous "six-pack" of well-developed abs? Finally, how about your thighs and calves? If you stand sideways and lower yourself partially in a half deep-knee bend, can you see any definition in your legs?

Make a mental note of what you see or, even better, write it down.

Step on the scale, preferable before breakfast in your underwear, barefoot, and at the same time and conditions each day. After noting your weight on the first day, go online and check your Body Mass Index (BMI), which is based on your height and weight. A BMI of 18.5 to 24.9 is normal, 25 to 29.5 is overweight, and 30 and higher is considered obese. Don't be upset if you are overweight or obese; two-thirds of American adults are, but make a commitment that you will work to get that weight down close to the normal range. It's important:

> ➤ According to the National Heart, Lung, and Blood Institute (2020), the higher a person's BMI, the greater the risk for diseases, including type 2 diabetes, heart disease, high blood pressure, respiratory problems, gallstones, and certain types of cancer.

Be patient: it took time to gain the extra weight, so it will take time to get rid of it. Your diet will play a key role along with exercise, so be sure to give the upcoming chapter on diet your fullest attention.

The tape measure is the last appearance and physical measurement benchmark, and like the scale, it is completely objective. It doesn't lie, exaggerate, or coddle you.

> ➤ Measure your waistline at the level between the top of your hip bones and naval, pulling the tape firmly but not too tight. Exhale just before you measure. Be aware that the measure for a man should not exceed 40 inches (102 cm), and for a woman, it's 35 inches (89 cm).

Beyond those measurement limits, professionals say there's too much belly fat, and that can interfere with numerous bodily functions. It also can possibly lead to the same diseases as an elevated BMI.

Benchmarking 2: Measuring Strength

The second phase of your benchmarking assessment is to see how much strength you have. A licensed physical trainer can run you through a series of measurements with different exercises and may even take a calculation of body fat and lean muscle percentages.

But you can take your own simple strength measurement by dropping down and seeing **how many push-ups** you can do. Start in a plank position, legs extended to the rear, arms fully extended shoulder-width apart, and your back level (no sagging or arching). Lower down fully so your nose or chest touches the floor, raise back up to the starting position, and repeat as many times as you can. Don't race: take about three seconds for each down-and-up cycle. Write down your total.

If you have access to a pull-up or chin-up bar, count **how many pull-ups** you can do (a pull-up is with your palms facing forward). Place your hands shoulder-width apart and pull up fully, lower all the way down ((not too fast), and repeat as many times as you can in good form (no half-ways). When you're done, write down the total. Or, if you can use dumbbells, determine the maximum weight you can curl eight to 10 times maximum. A curl is raising the dumbbells from the arms-lowered position up to your shoulders, then slowly lowering back down.

As your weight training program progresses, you can periodically repeat these exercises and measure your improvements.

Fitness, Health, Longevity

Your motivation to get into, or get *back* into, weightlifting and other exercises to gain strength in middle-age is based, at least in part, on how you want to look and feel. You want to see a well-built body in the mirror with visibly larger, defined muscles and a flatter gut. You want to feel the muscles expanding under your skin at the end of your workouts as blood rushes to the hard-working muscle cells and fibers in the "pumping iron" effect. You want more energy, more bounce to your step, more endurance to keep you going longer. You want to look and feel fit. You want to be stronger.

These are the motivating factors that will get you started on your weight and strength-building program. They hopefully will be enough to keep you going because achieving your fitness goals will take time and effort.

To further reinforce your commitment, let's pick up on what was mentioned above in the discussion of benchmarking: the health aspects of getting in shape and staying in shape, and getting your weight down and keeping it down.

More Life to Your Years

There's an expression that was popular among long-distance runners and has spread to the weightlifting and fitness community overall:

> ➤ "Working out and staying in shape will add more life to your years and may even add more years to your life."

In other words, your commitment to building muscle and getting into good cardiovascular condition definitely will make every day richer and more vibrant and may also help you to live longer. All in all, that's not a bad deal. It gives you something to work for, to invest time and energy in, and stay with over the long term.

According to the Mayo Clinic (2020), regular exercise can improve health and manage the symptoms of chronic illnesses that are long-term, limit activities, and interfere with a normal lifestyle. Given the importance of exercise in preventing heart disease, it is covered separately in the following section.

Everyday activities. Strength training with weightlifting not only improves muscle strength and increases endurance, but makes daily activities easier to do and slows the decline in muscle strength related to disease. Every day, we are lifting, carrying, standing, walking, crouching, bending, and generally challenging our muscles, joints, bones, and tendons as well as pushing our circulatory and respiratory systems as we work our hearts and lungs during exertion. The better the state of our physical condition, the easier the work we do will be, and when we're in good shape, we feel better.

Joint stability. Flexibility exercises can help you regain an optimal range of motion by providing stability to your joints to enhance their functionality, and the risk of falls can be reduced with stability exercises. Weightlifting and other resistance exercises, when done correctly, will increase stability and flexibility and will further help by strengthening the muscles that support the joints. For example, by strengthening the quadriceps muscles at the front of our thighs, we can help control the kneecap and knee socket, preventing excess motions that can wear away the cartilage that lubricates and cushions the knees.

Diabetes. Regular exercise can lower the risk of adult-onset type 2 diabetes by enabling insulin to lower blood sugar levels more effectively. For those already with type 2 diabetes, resistance exercise with weightlifting, along with aerobics, can reduce the risk of heart disease.

Type 2 diabetes is often associated with obesity, so the weight reduction benefits of exercise can directly reduce the risks and symptoms of diabetes.

Weight control. Physical activity can help you control your weight and boost your energy because weightlifting burns calories as does cardiovascular training. However, exercise alone does not optimize weight loss; it is the combination of diet and exercise that is most effective. In a later chapter, we'll examine how diet and exercise combined can make the greatest effects in getting those excess pounds off and keeping them off.

Arthritis. Exercise has been found t0 reduce joint pain, maintain muscle strength in arthritis-affected joints, and reduce stiffness in joints, resulting in improved quality of life and physical function even for those who have been suffering from arthritis for years. Those with arthritis symptoms should choose low-impact exercise. Any weightlifting that puts extra pressure on joints may require modifying certain movements to reduce the strain.

Asthma. The heavy, deeper breathing associated with weightlifting and all intensive exercise appears to help reduce the severity and frequency of asthma attacks. The depth of breathing during exercise, combined with increased blood circulation and oxygen delivery, may strengthen the lungs and air sacs where oxygen is transferred to the bloodstream. The deep breathing performed during intense exercise also strengthens the diaphragm muscle, which controls breathing by facilitating inhaling and exhaling.

Back pain. Abdominal and core-challenging resistance exercises strengthen the muscles around your spine, and these exercises may help reduce back pain symptoms. Also, low-impact aerobic exercises, performed regularly, are believed to increase strength and endurance in the back and improve the function of the lumbar and thoracic back muscles. We'll cover stretching and flexibility routines later that can ease your sore lower back in just a few minutes.

Bone density. Our bones are porous, which is normal. But as we enter middle-age, this porosity can increase, and the bones become less dense, more brittle, and more susceptible to breakage. This condition is called osteoporosis.

Falls are a common cause of bone fractures, but there are others, too, including some that are exercise-induced. Running or jumping on a hard surface, for example, may cause small stress fractures, which are hairline cracks in the bones that can cause pain and lead to larger breaks. The right kinds of exercise, however, can help reverse osteoporosis and make bones stronger:

> **High-impact**, weight-bearing exercises include activities like dancing, jumping rope, running and jogging outdoors (with proper athletic shoes to prevent injury), hiking (especially uphill), and playing tennis or racquetball.

> **Low-impact,** weight-bearing exercises may be better for those already diagnosed with osteoporosis and include working out on elliptical machines or stair climbers and walking at a brisk moderate pace either outdoors or on a treadmill.

> **Muscle-strengthening** exercises include weightlifting with free weights, like dumbbells and kettle weights, or weight machines with cable-pulled weights, stretching elastic exercise bands, or performing bodyweight calisthenics.

> **Flexibility** exercises can involve stretching (especially after a workout), yoga, and Pilates. Yoga is especially recognized for improving flexibility and balance, which can help prevent falls. If you already have osteoporosis concerns, it's a good idea to check with your doctor or a trained professional physical therapist to make sure you are not straining body parts that are at risk.

Mental health. Exercise reduces symptoms of two of the most common mental and emotional concerns: anxiety and depression. Both of these conditions are frequently caused by stress, which triggers the body's sympathetic response, the well-known "fight or flight" reaction to perceived dangers. The body gets ready for action with elevated heart and breathing rates as well as the release of the energy hormones, adrenaline, and cortisol. In this charged state, anxiety can occur, and when it is continuous over time or chronic, it can lead to autoimmune responses, including chronic inflammation.

> Resistance or cardiovascular exercise takes advantage of the body's state of readiness by effectively putting energy hormones to work and burning the extra glycogen they have sent to your muscles. When the workout is over, and you have cooled down, heart and breathing rates return to normal. The workout also will release beta-endorphin hormones that give you a feeling of elation, and the anxiety can be dissipated.

➤ Depression can occur when the parasympathetic response, which cools things down, overdoes it, reducing normal energy levels and depressing the central nervous system. As with anxiety, beta-endorphin hormones can give the person a sense of elation, and the depressive state can be reduced or eliminated.

➤ Caveat: Chronic anxiety and depression may not respond sufficiently to exercise, meditation, or yoga, and in those cases, professional care may be necessary.

Dementia. Cognition disorders, especially in people with dementia, may be reduced by exercise. Moreover, those not currently suffering from dementia, and who are physically active regularly with resistance and aerobic exercises, are at reduced risk of developing cognitive impairment and dementia or appreciably slowing its onset.

Cancer. Can the right exercise routines prevent cancer? There is evidence, as the Mayo Clinic reports, that exercise can lower the risk of dying from prostate, breast, and colorectal cancer, and exercise may also help reduce the likelihood of developing other forms of cancer. Exercise may also improve the quality of life and overall fitness for those who have recovered from cancer. Many doctors believe that exercise's role in lowering weight and reducing the likelihood of other diseases keeps the immune system strong, and this helps prevent cancer cells from proliferating, forming tumors, or metastasizing (spreading).

Heart Health

The prevention of heart disease is closely associated with exercise, and with good reason. Exercise can play an important role in preventing heart disease or reducing its risks. Both of the major categories of exercise, resistance and cardiovascular, when performed for sufficient time and with sufficient intensity, can improve overall heart healthiness and contribute to the prevention of heart attacks, heart failure, and strokes.

Heart disease includes atherosclerosis, the build-up of plaque in the coronary arteries that supply the heart with oxygen-rich blood. Over time, as the plaque accumulates, the flow of blood to the heart becomes restricted. Early warnings include angina pectoris, which is a pain in the chest during exercise. Preventing or limiting the build-up of plaque is directly related to controlling the levels of blood lipids.

Can exercise lower blood lipids? The results of studies are encouraging within limits. Blood lipids include HDL (good) cholesterol, which is credited with carrying away LDL (bad) cholesterol, the low density, sponge-like blood lipid which can add to the plaque that clogs arteries, leading to atherosclerosis or coronary heart disease.

Another major blood lipid group is triglycerides, which are fats that circulate in the bloodstream and also can lead to heart disease.

Studies that show exercise-induced reductions of LDL cholesterol and triglycerides and elevated beneficial HDL cholesterol indicate that the **intensity of the exercise is a key factor.** Whether it's weightlifting or aerobics, the workout needs to get the heart rate up and keep it up for at least 25 to 40 minutes three or more times per week.

Controlling hypertension. Exercise can also contribute to lowering hypertension, or high blood pressure, which is a primary cause of strokes.

➤ Exercise and high blood pressure are connected because your heart grows stronger with regular, consistent physical activity. When your heart is stronger, it can pump more blood volume with less exertion. As a result of your heart working less to pump blood, your blood pressure is lowered as the pressure on your arteries is reduced.

➤ Exercise has been clinically proven to lower systolic blood pressure (the first number in your blood pressure reading) by four to nine millimeters of mercury (mm Hg). So, with the right exercise, a systolic pressure of 135 could be lowered to 126, which is within the normal range, and about the same result as from some blood pressure prescription drugs. As a result, for some who have hypertension, regular exercise can reduce or replace a dependency on blood pressure medication.

➤ The benefits of exercise extend to those whose blood pressure is at normal levels, which is less than 130/80 mm Hg. Exercise can help keep your blood pressure from rising as you grow older. Helping you to keep your weight down and maintain a normal BMI is another way exercise helps you to control blood pressure.

Resistance training has also been demonstrated to help protect cardiovascular health. In *BMC Public Health* (2012), researchers reported that the combination of resistance and aerobic exercise was effective in helping people lose more weight and fat than either of these exercise techniques alone as well as creating increased overall cardiovascular fitness.

➤ The lipid-lowering benefits of resistance training for people with high overall cholesterol were cited in the medical journal *Atherosclerosis* (2011), showing that those who performed resistance training cleared LDL cholesterol from their bloodstream faster than those who did not train.

High-intensity interval training is generally safe and effective for most people and can take less time. In high-intensity interval training, you alternate exercising at high levels of intensity and exercising at a less intense level for short periods. Even activities such as walking at higher intensities count.

Low-intensity exercise is valuable for helping to lower your weight and to relieve stress, and some studies suggest that even walking at a moderate pace for 150 minutes a week can have positive cardiovascular and overall health benefits. This intensity and duration is an alternative to the frequently recommended 75 minutes per week of intense exercise.

Post-coronary exercise is generally recommended to aid recovery and strengthen the heart, which is a muscle, and like all muscles. benefits from regular exercise. In these cases, the type and intensity of the exercise should be medically supervised.

Now, let's move on to Chapter 2 and see how you can build muscles at age 40, 50, and beyond.

Chapter 2:

Build Muscles at 40, 50, and Beyond

Are you skeptical? Do you think that the years have gone by and that you should have gotten into weightlifting and bodybuilding 10 years ago, or even 20 or more years ago? Or you worked out with weights back then, but your career got in the way, and you quit? Those years may be gone, but your opportunity to build those muscles, and gain that strength, is still here, waiting only for you to say to yourself, "This is my chance to make up for lost time and build the body I've always wanted."

Consider when Tug McGraw said, "Ya gotta believe," the admonition that turned around the losing New York Mets, and put them into the 1974 World Series. It's all about positive thinking and having confidence in yourself.

It's not too late. Even if you are middle-aged and have never worked out, even if you're overweight, out of shape, and lack energy, it is not too late for you. This is your time if you have the motivation and commitment to start and continue a weightlifting program. If you are ready, you can fulfill your hopes and dreams of fitness, health, and energy. *Yes, you can* lift serious weights and build serious lean muscles. You can do this.

The Science of Muscle-Building

To reinforce your confidence and erase any doubts you may have about whether it is possible to become a successful weightlifter at this time in your life, this chapter is going to give you the basics from science and experience to convince you that there are physiological processes that you can initiate that will pay you back generously with results that will surprise you, maybe even astound you.

Science may not be the first thing that comes to mind when planning a muscle-building program, but it is important to ignore the old clichés and anecdotal tales because safely and effectively building lean muscles is based entirely on scientific principles. What does this mean? The scientific method means facts are established by test results that can be consistently repeated and not by opinions and traditions. The principles that apply to young weightlifters also apply to middle-age weightlifters with the understanding that age requires some adjustments to achieve good results safely.

The Concept of Hypertrophy

The muscles we are concerned with are the 650 skeletal muscles that enable us to move and do work. They are made up of muscle fibers which, in turn, are built up from fine thread-like fibers called sarcomeres and myofibrils. These muscle fibers are the fundamental elements of muscular contraction. When you flex a muscle or put it to work, it is within the fibers where the action is taking place. Keep these fibers in mind as we progress because they will be the units of growth that strengthen and build your muscles.

Muscles contract on command when certain nerves, called motor neurons, receive their signals from cells known as the sarcoplasmic reticulum. As your body becomes more conditioned, the signals will become more adept at getting your muscles to contract, and you will become stronger even before muscles are much larger. If you can train to activate your motor neurons effectively, it can jumpstart the processes to build bigger muscles to lift heavier weights. We'll explain this in greater detail in the instructional chapters.

First, do the damage. The process of hypertrophy, the creation of muscle growth, begins with the damage done to muscle fibers during weightlifting. The extreme effort of lifting or pulling heavy weights breaks down some of the muscle fibers that are involved in the hard work; this occurs at the cellular level and is completely normal. Your cells are being sacrificed by doing more work than they are accustomed to.

Next, repair the damage. To repair the damage, the cells use amino acid molecules to fuse into muscle fibers and to form new myofibrils out of strands of protein. This is why protein needs to be an important component of a weightlifter's diet; it is the building block from which the myofibrils are constructed.

Importantly, during this process of hypertrophy:

➤ The myofibrils are not just repaired and rebuilt to their previous size but are made thicker and more numerous. They get slightly larger. They experience growth.

➤ Hypertrophy, or muscle growth, occurs when the production of muscle protein exceeds the previous pre-damage level. On a day-to-day basis, the muscle tissue increments are microscopic, but over time they accumulate, and muscle bulk becomes visible.

Satellite cells. The effectiveness of your hypertrophy is dependent upon what are known as satellite cells, which spur the growth of the myofibrils by increasing muscle protein nuclei and enabling the cells to divide more frequently. According to trainer and coach John Leyva, who is technical editor of the *BuiltLean Blog* (2020), the degree to which the satellite cells are active is dependent on the type and resistance of the exercises performed and the amount of stress that is placed on the muscles:

1. **Tension of the muscles** is the result of progressively increasing the load that muscles are lifting and pulling, exceeding the amount of resistance they are accustomed to. So if you do bicep curls regularly with 15-pound dumbbells, your biceps and upper arms will retain their current muscle size and strength, but will not grow larger or stronger until you increase the weight to introduce greater resistance and cause stress.

2. **Damage to muscle cells** and tissues releases immune system cells and inflammatory molecules that trigger the activation of satellite cells which, in turn, stimulate the growth of muscle tissue protein and boost hypertrophy. One clear signal that this has occurred is muscle soreness in the hours and even days after your workout. This is due to the damage done during the workout, and it sets the stage for the over-rebuilding of muscle tissue to follow. Much of the soreness is from lactic acid buildup which will dissipate within a day or two.

3. **Metabolic stress** results from intense muscle tension and causes swelling of the cells in and around the muscle. It's the result of the accumulation of blood, which is bringing extra oxygen to the tensed and damaged muscle fibers, plus the arrival of glycogen, the sugar molecules that provide the muscle cells with energy. These effects

may contribute to increased rebuilding, but much of the increased muscle size after the workout, while impressive, is temporary, and the muscles will return to their normal size as the fluids drain from the muscles.

Hormones

The role of hormones in building muscles is frequently debated. This is what is known today about the natural hormones in our bodies:

➤ Testosterone and insulin-like growth factor I (IGH-I) are the two most active hormones that contribute to muscle growth.

➤ While testosterone is at higher levels in men, women also have testosterone (and men also have estrogen), although a woman's testosterone is at a lower level, which is a key reason that men can build muscles more readily than women.

➤ Both men and women can increase strength through weightlifting and other resistance exercises.

While most of our testosterone is not free-roaming or available to affect muscle building, studies show that hard resistance exercise can release more testosterone, which can activate satellite cells, prevent or reduce protein breakdown, increase protein synthesis, and stimulate other anabolic hormones. It may also encourage muscle cell receptors to be more sensitive to free testosterone. Testosterone can also increase the number of neurotransmitters at the site of damaged fiber, help activate tissue growth, and stimulate growth hormone responses.

The bottom line on natural hormones in our bodies is that resistance training can stimulate the release of hormones that further enhance the building of muscle and strength.

Hormones supplements? You are not encouraged to take hormone supplements to build muscle mass unless prescribed by a doctor following a blood test that identifies a hormone deficiency.

Rest and Muscle Loss vs. Muscle Gain

The muscle repairs and rebuilding we've been discussing do not occur during the time while you are actually lifting the weights and damaging the muscle fibers. Instead, muscle growth — hypertrophy — takes place while you, and your muscles, are at rest.

It is during rest that recovery can take place. If the muscles continue to be worked, even to less extreme levels, there will be no opportunity for hypertrophy to do its work and, at best, no repairs can occur. Of greater concern, hard resistance exercise performed too soon after a good weightlifting session can have negative effects:

➤ If your muscles do not receive sufficient rest to prepare and conduct their repairs, you can reverse the protein-building process and allow your body to fall into a destructive or catabolic state. Over time, this can lead to muscle loss.

➤ The time needed for recovery and hypertrophy after a resistance exercise session is about 24 to 48 hours. So weightlifting that challenges any specific muscle group should not work that same muscle group for at least one day, preferably two days.

➤ If you follow a routine of doing total-body resistance workouts in a single workout session, then you should not have weightlifting or resistance sessions more than three times a week.

Weightlifters over 40. The need for rest and recovery is of special importance to you as a middle-age weightlifter because your recovery time is longer as a function of your age and a slower metabolism. A two-day rest and recovery period after each weightlifting session is ideal for you.

Up the protein. During the rest and recovery days, your diet should be rich in protein since the amino acids that make up protein molecules are needed for the repair of muscle fibers. We'll cover everything you need to know about diet in a later chapter, but for now, assume that you will want to have more meat, fish, dairy, and eggs, all of which are high in complete protein.

Vegetarians and vegans can increase their consumption of beans and other legumes, plus soybeans, buckwheat, and quinoa, which are among the few plant sources of complete protein, including the nine essential amino acids that our bodies need to get from our food.

Over 40: It's Not Too Late

We've just been through the scientific basis for muscle building, and you can appreciate there is no magic or mystery involved. Resistance exercises, followed by adequate rest and recovery and with enough protein in the diet, will build muscles. The cells that compose your muscles get damaged, then repair themselves with added protein, and the cells then over-repair.

As a result, lean muscle tissue increases in size over time, and you grow stronger. Hypertrophy is inevitable if the rules of the game are followed.

Yes, you may be thinking that may work for the young, but you are over 40, or maybe over 50 or 60, and yet now you are being told that it's not too late for you to get those muscles bigger and stronger.

How can this be? With age, your muscles are not as large, some body fat has accumulated, energy isn't the same, and your knees, shoulders, and other joints ache when you bend, crouch, or lift something. Your testosterone level has undoubtedly slipped lower. The porosity of your bones may have increased, maybe osteoporosis is happening, and your bones may be more susceptible to breakage.

An Ideal Time

So, you may ask, all in all, is this really a good time to start, or get back into, serious weightlifting and other forms of resistance exercises? Isn't it too late?

Not only is it not too late, as you have already read, but it's also an ideal time. Stronger, bigger muscles are not a vanity. They are your protection against growing weaker, frail, fragile, less mobile, less flexible, and, here's the big one, less likely to be overweight or obese, and subject to heart disease, diabetes, and a long list of other serious diseases. It's your time right now. You have nothing to lose, and everything — health, longevity, strength, energy and vitality, a great build you can be proud of, self-esteem — to gain.

Weightlifting coach and trainer TC Luomo sums it up in his *TC Nation* (2019) article by asking if you were an aging professional athlete, presumably having passed age 40, and didn't have what you used to, and you weren't keeping up with the younger athletes, would you give up, retire, and get soft, or would you work harder to regain what you've lost? More to the point, if you wanted to play even better now, even if your joints ache a bit and you're less flexible than before, would you train and work out harder or easier now? His answer is "Harder, of course."

You, at age 40-plus, have unquestionably lost some of the luxuries of your youth so it becomes necessary to train harder — and smarter — to compensate for what the years have taken, gradually and unseen, as a normal part of the aging process. But when you were born, as TC Luomo puts it, you did not have a 40-year expiration date tattooed on your posterior, so what's to stop you from getting back into the muscle-building and fitness game and doing it better than ever before?

New Rules of the Training Game

If training hard and training smart is the formula for success after age 40, there is a set of rules, let's call them guidelines, that will get you where you need to go faster, easier, and more effectively than picking up a barbell, pulling, a cable, stretching a rubber exercise band, or dropping into the plank position and knocking off some push-ups.

The following chapters will guide you through the specific exercises, but these guidelines are meant to give you the big picture, the perspective, on what to do and why to do it.

> ➤ Quick definition: Reps are repetition, the number of times you lift or pull the weight successively. In total, the repetitions become one set. So an upper-arm workout might be three sets of eight reps of barbell curls, with a one-minute rest between sets.

1. Breathe deeply. Unless you have been working hard on the cardiovascular side and have been running, race walking, cycling, swimming, or hitting the elliptical machine or stair climber with sufficient frequency and intensity, you are probably not close to a high level of aerobic conditioning. OK, you may think, "I get it, for cardiovascular health and to help keep off the pounds, I need to deal with that, but later, because I want to get going with weightlifting first."

Yes, the long-term benefits of cardio training are fantastic, but this is about getting you in shape for the immediate term, to ensure that you have the aerobic capacity to breathe and function as you lift weights. This aerobic training will involve three or four days a week when you perform your resistance exercises and will take 10 to 20 minutes starting out. Don't force your heart rate up in the beginning, just be sure that you warm up slowly for two or three minutes. Pick up the pace so that you are breathing hard and deeply for a minute, slow down for one minute, then pick up the pace again and give it a good intensity for one minute, slow again, then fast again. End with a one-minute slowdown.

> ➤ This is an abbreviated version of HIIT, or high-intensity interval training, a compressed form of aerobic conditioning. It will save you the time of slower, dragged-out exercise, and has been proven to increase the growth and vibrancy of mitochondria, the energy factories in our muscle cells.

> ➤ Perform this aerobic exercise *before* you begin the weightlifting, not after. Your objective is to oxygenate your muscle cells before the stress that the resistance exercises create. It is also better to get your heart muscle warmed up slowly rather than forcing it up suddenly with eight reps of lifting a heavy weight.

2. Work hard. Whether you prefer to lift heavy or lighter weights, you are going to be working hard.

You may be lifting heavier weights with fewer reps because some professionals believe it is the best way to catch you up with where you left off, or where you need to start if this is all new to you. That is not to say that you'll be straining, but the recommendations from many trainers are to forget about doing lots of reps with light weights. They say lighter weights with lots of reps may help build endurance but won't address the building of muscle mass or strength.

There is an opposite approach also advocated by some trainers: lifting lighter weights and doing more reps. For example, instead of doing eight to 10 reps with a heavy weight, you lift a lighter weight for 15 to 20 reps. The advantage of lighter weights is that they place less strain on joints, tendons, and ligaments, and since each of us responds uniquely to physical effort and stress, you will need to be the final judge of what works best for you. The following chapters will cover the various exercises and workout routines you can perform.

3. Manage the pain. The expression, "No pain, no gain," became popular in the 1980s when the weightlifting and calisthenics movements began to gain momentum. This expression was subsequently criticized for encouraging people to push past their limits which could lead to injuries ranging from torn ligaments and muscles to joint damage. Today, we know that the responsible approach is to push towards your limits but don't exceed them. Pain is a warning and should not be ignored.

Lifting heavy weights can cause a variety of pains. Joints can creak and ache, muscles can cry out when pushed hard as you try to get that last rep done to conclude a set. These are generally normal but only within limits. Give that last rep a good effort but force it. Do your best but don't punish yourself.

> ➢ Be especially careful with your shoulders because that set of muscles, called the rotator cuff, is susceptible to tears if subject to shock or excessive stress. Most of your skeletal muscles will hurt too much for you to damage them, and the pain will force you to back off or stop the movement, but your shoulders give little warning when at risk.

4. Heavy, but not too heavy. Some weightlifters practice powerlifting, which is very few reps with very heavy weights. This not for you since your 40-plus-year-old joints and connective tissues no longer have the flexibility and resilience they had 20 years ago. So, if you prefer to lift heavy weights, make sure that the weight is not so heavy that you can't do at least eight reps without difficulty. If you can only do three or four reps, the weight is too heavy. Ratchet back until you can find a weight that you max out at eight to 10 reps.

Remember, building muscle and strength takes time and patience. So does losing the extra weight you may be hoping to shed. That's again why the motivation to get started is not enough; you need to commit to going the distance, putting in the months and then making it part of your lifestyle for the years ahead.

5. Rest, but not too much. By now, the importance of rest and recovery time has been driven home; you got it, muscles get damaged and need time to build, rebuild, and overbuild. Hypertrophy requires rest. The right amount for the age 40-plus weightlifter is 48 hours. Those two days are what your body needs to get the muscles rebuilt and ready for action. One day of rest might have been enough when you were younger, but at this stage of life, that extra time is needed. If you rush back to the weights too soon, as you have learned earlier in this chapter, more harm than good can occur.

But there is a limit. Too much rest allows the muscles to get lazy, to forget the conditioning, and start to soften. So two or three days of rest between weightlifting sessions is perfect, four or five days is stretching it a bit, and six or more days rest is too much. Never worry about one missed scheduled workout day, but have the self-discipline to catch up sooner rather than later. Each workout is like an investment, and you want to protect it.

Now, let's head to Chapter 3, which deals with how much weight you should lift.

Chapter 3:

How Much You Should Lift

There are two distinctive camps when it comes to the "how much" question: how much weight should a person who is middle-aged be lifting? One side says you should lift heavier weights with fewer reps per set, and the other side advocates taking it easier with the weight and giving the effort more reps. For example, should you lift a 50-pound barbell eight to 10 times to complete one set, or lift a 2-pound barbell 16 to 20 times per set? What about greater extremes, like a 9-pound weight for a maximum of just two reps, or doing 30 to 40 reps with a 12- to 15-pound barbell?

Avoid extremes. For reasons of safety and effectiveness, we can toss out the extremes. As you'll recall from the previous discussion, lifting a weight that you can only raise cleanly and correctly one, two, or at most three times is definitely not recommended for anyone over age 40 whose joints, ligaments, and tendons are no longer as flexible and resilient as when the person was 20 years younger. The other extreme of lifting very light weights for 30 or more times in a set is also not recommended because while it may be safe and not likely to cause injury, the results in building muscle and strength will be minimal.

Between the extremes, there are more moderate alternatives; one that emphasizes building muscle mass and increasing strength, and one which provides benefits of endurance and muscle toning with less risk of injury or strain.

The Heavier Weight Options

The word "heavy" has different meanings to different people and in different situations. A 10-pound weight can be considered heavy if you are holding it at arm's length, but light if you are lifting a 10-pound barbell. When it comes to how heavy the weights you lift should be, it's a matter of the desired result, safety, and degrees of intensity.

Moderately Heavy Weights

Advocates of what we'll call the *moderately heavier weight* approach believe that just because you are a middle-aged weightlifter does not prevent you from lifting heavy weights. If your goal is to develop lean, well-defined muscle mass in the shortest amount of time, moderate heavier weights are the right weights for you. Advocates' experiences lead to the conclusion that the right weight and number of reps per set offer optimal muscle-building results, safely, without over demanding joints and connective tissues.

How heavy? It's easy to determine your safe level of moderately heavier weights at any time in your progress cycle because as you get stronger, the amount you can lift increases in direct proportion to your capacity:

> ➤ Your capacity is based on the number of reps you can do within a range of weights with eight to 10 reps being the optimal number in a set.

This means you can lift the first six or seven reps without difficulty, but number eight, nine, or at most 10, are barely doable. You should be able to get to this level, but no higher. You will need to make this calculation for each weightlifting exercise: arms, shoulders, chest, upper body, core and abdominals, back, and legs so that the workout for each muscle group is optimized. If you can only perform five, six, or seven reps, the weight is too heavy, and if you can get past 10 reps, the weight is too light.

You will need to increase the weight level periodically as your strength increases, and when you reach the time when the weight that was tough to raise fully at the eighth to 10th rep is no longer as tough, and you can now do more reps. If the weight can be lifted or pulled more than 10 times, it's time to increase the resistance, not the reps. Be sure that while you are lifting and counting the reps, you are performing the movements by keeping in good form: no jerking, or half-lifts.

Ultra-Heavy vs. Moderately Heavy Weights

You may be wondering about powerlifting. Many seasoned, successful weightlifters believe, unshakably, that for both men and women, the ideal method to build muscle mass is to lift very heavy weights and to increase the weight consistently over time. On the extreme end of this perspective, competitive bodybuilders and powerlifters perform very low reps (from one to three at most) lifting extremely heavy weights, which are 90 percent to 100 percent of the maximum they can lift in one single rep. At the least, bodybuilding and strength optimization is a deep passion for these weightlifters, and to some, it's how they make a living so evidently they do what works.

Why does this ultra-heavy lifting work? Clinical studies in laboratories show that lifting heavier weight, for example, at least 70 percent of a person's maximum one-rep weight activates "fast-twitch type 2 muscle fibers, which play a key role in developing muscle strength and encouraging hypertrophy, which is the process of increasing the size of muscle fiber cells.

But there is a downside. While type 2 muscle fibers may gain more power, they are also subject to early fatigue, and muscle fiber stimulation depends on the duration of how long they are under tension from resistance. If the muscle fibers are not under sufficient tension for enough time, they will be less able to effectively initiate hypertrophy.

Of even greater importance, *ultra-heavy weights are not recommended* for middle-age weightlifters. It only takes one rep of a very heavy weight to pull or tear a muscle, tendon, or ligament.

This means that for you, at age 40-plus, moderately heavy weights are preferable to ultra-heavy weights:

> ➤ Because of concerns over ultra-heavy lifting, many aspiring weightlifters are achieving success with the moderately heavy approach: eight to 10 reps at between 70 percent and 75 percent of the maximum you can lift one time. (No need to bring a calculator to the workout; determine the weight you can perform at least eight reps but no more than 10 reps; that is your ideal moderately heavy weight target.)

The Lighter Weight Option

Now let's consider the alternative to lifting heavier weights at the other extreme: many reps with weights (or resistance) you can lift many more times before reaching your maximum effort. We know that lighter weights are less risky since they place less stress on the joints, muscles, tendons, and ligaments. But can lighter weights build the larger, more defined muscles you want and measurably increase your strength?

More is Less

These are the effects when you increase the number of your reps into a higher range, like at least 15 reps per set or even 20 or more. Some who favor lighter weights may lift as many as 32 reps before calling it quits in the set. The specific weight you can manage when doing many reps is estimated to be roughly 50 percent to 60 percent of the maximum you can lift just one time, a single rep. Determination of your ideal lighter weight is similar to moderately heavier weights, but now it's finding out the maximum weight you can lift about 20 to 24 times consecutively.

➢ You may feel like you worked hard after 24 reps, and you have! But the research indicates that you have not lifted a sufficient amount of weight to trigger a type 2, fast-twitch response, which is what is needed to promote big muscle growth.

But workouts involving higher reps and lower weights have their own set of benefits because they activate different muscle fibers, called type 1, or "slow-twitch muscle fibers. These responses may not build much muscle and create less power than type 2 responses, but they do increase endurance and are slower to fatigue.

In consequence, a workout with lighter weights and many more reps will not necessarily increase your strength but will build muscular endurance. You will burn more calories with higher reps because these longer workouts help burn fat as well as carbohydrates, thus reducing your total body fat level which can result in a leaner, toned appearance. Your post-workout feeling will be more of a glow, and you will be less likely to experience the pain of working out with heavier weights.

Summing up: In considering whether to go for lifting lighter weights and doing more reps or lifting moderately heavy weights with fewer reps, there are positives to each:

➢ With lighter weights and more reps, you will not build muscle or strength compared to lifting moderately heavier weights, but you will increase muscular endurance, and your risk of joint, ligament, tendon, or muscle damage is lower.

➤ Lifting moderately heavy weights will get you to your muscle-building and strength-increasing goals, but be aware there is a higher risk of strain or injury. Be careful not to overdo the weights, and let the number of reps be your guide. If you can't lift the weight eight times, it's too heavy.

Middle-Age Celebrity Weightlifters

Becoming a weightlifter after age 40, or returning to weightlifting at this age after a long hiatus, is not something new or unique. On the contrary, men and women who do not want to accept the negative consequences of maturity, who want to slow the aging process and maintain good health, are working out with weights in health clubs, fitness centers, gyms, and at home. Their routines may vary from individual to individual, but they are united in the common goals of wanting to be stronger, and to look stronger.

Middle-agers working out and increasing their musculature, getting stronger, and shaping up is going on all around us, and a visit to a fitness center will confirm that it's not just younger people but many of us of all ages who are curling dumbbells, lifting barbells, swinging kettle weights, pulling cables, stretching exercise bands, and doing pull-ups. The treadmills, ellipticals, and cycles are frequently occupied by older men and women who are including a good cardiovascular workout in their routines.

To give you other examples of middle-age weightlifting and physical fitness advocates, we can turn to some action-hero celebrities for inspiration: Jason Statham, Daniel Craig, Dwayne "The Rock" Johnson, and Hugh Jackman.

Jason Statham

Jason Statham's films include *The Mechanic, Furious 7, Death Race*, and *Hobbs and Shaw*. In these and many other films and shows, we know him as an action hero scaling buildings, overcoming adversaries, and being an all-around tough guy. But Jason is no kid, and at age 52, he's working out most days of the week as hard as he ever has, reminiscent of his younger days when he was a diver and footballer. That is why he maintains an enviable physique and looks and feels like his younger self.

What's his routine? Jason's objectives are to preserve lean muscle, get rid of any extra body fat, and stay strong and flexible. He wants to keep his metabolism from slowing down, and he attributes his fitness to his diet as much as his workouts. We'll cover diet in a later chapter, but here are the highlights of what he eats.

A responsible diet. Jason follows what appears to be close to the Mediterranean diet, which focuses on oats and other whole grains, nuts and seeds, cold-water fish (high in omega 3 antioxidants), lean chicken, brown rice, lots of fresh fruit, and a variety of vegetables. Protein is a priority to keep building muscle. He believes that about 95 percent of his diet is healthy, though he allows himself some chocolate (dark chocolate is now recognized as beneficial, so no guilt needed). To his credit and nutritional advantage, he avoids greasy fried foods (as everyone concerned about their health should do).

You will see a full day of Jason's nutritional selections in Chapter 6, but here are the highlights to give you the idea of what makes a great diet for a middle-age athlete who wants to get stronger, stay fit, and keep healthy:

➤ **Breakfast** begins with fresh fruits, including strawberries and pineapple, followed by oatmeal, which is loaded with cholesterol-reducing fiber, then a good protein hit with poached eggs.

➤ **Lunch** often includes brown rice, which provides quality carbohydrates, fiber, vitamins, minerals, and some protein. Jason adds steamed vegetables for added nutrition; this combination is actually a vegan lunch which he thinks is good on occasion. He often adds a bowl of hot miso soup, which Jason thinks is delicious and healthy (it is but be aware of the sodium level if you're concerned about hypertension).

➤ **Snack** time is nut time in the form of the cashews, almonds, and walnuts he likes to crunch on. Nuts also come into play with peanut butter, but not the processed, sugar-loaded commercial brands. Jason stays with the unprocessed, all-natural version which is ground peanuts and nothing else. (Again, a head's up on salt; salt-free is better for you.

➤ **Dinner** is the heavier protein meal with lean beef one night, chicken or fish on another. Salmon or other cold-water fish are the healthiest for you, and try to keep the chicken lean. Jason's evening meal includes both vegetables and a leafy green salad.

(Hint: Start the evening meal with a large green salad, and you'll eat less of the higher calorie foods to follow.)

An awesome workout. Here's one day of a seven-day workout that Jason performs. This is his workout, not yours, so be inspired to work towards it someday. More practically, say to yourself that if he can do all that powerlifting, what you will be learning in the following chapter is pretty easy by comparison. Remember, Jason Statham has been working out with increasing intensity all life, so don't feel you're not measuring up. If Jason was just starting on his exercise program at middle-age or getting back to weightlifting after a 15- or 20-year hiatus, he'd probably be following the same program you'll be following. Here's his actual Day 1:

Deadlift One-Rep Max Progression

This involves a series of warm-ups and one-rep bench press exercises, paving the way for a solitary goal: the almighty deadlift (i.e., a one-repetition max of the heaviest weight you can lift at one time).

As a warm-up to get the blood circulating and oxygenate the muscles, Jason first hops on the rowing machine and rows for 10 minutes at a moderate pace. Then, a pyramid circuit in which he does one rep of each of these three: barbell squat, press-up (same as push-up), and ring pull-ups using a light weight and his bodyweight. One round of the circuit is done, then repeated but with two reps; pause, again each one for three reps, then four, then five reps. Then he descends the circuit with four reps, three, two, and finally one rep.

So now Jason is warmed up and ready to go to work. If you feel exhausted just reading about his warm-up, fasten your seatbelt for what's about to follow.

Jason Statham's deadlift workout is the ultra-heavy weightlifting we discussed in the previous section, and it was agreed it is not for you. But Jason has his agenda, and here it is. A deadlift is the buzzword for the one-rep maximum weight routine. You will see he starts heavy, gets heavier, then gets really heavy, maxing out at 365 pounds. Here is Jason's deadlift sequence for the barbell squat:

1. 10 reps lifting 135 pounds, followed by one-minute rest.
2. 5 reps lifting 185 pounds, followed by two-minute rest.
3. 3 reps lifting 235 pounds, followed by three-minute rest.
4. 2 reps lifting 285 pounds, followed by three-minute rest.

5. 1 rep lifting 325 pounds, followed by three-minute rest.
6. 1 rep lifting 350 pounds, followed by three-minute rest.
7. 1 rep lifting 360 pounds, followed by three-minute rest.
8. 1 rep lifting 365 pounds, followed by three-minute rest, then cool down.

Cool down for Jason is doing footwork on a trampoline for 10 minutes; an alternative could be 10 to 15 minutes on a treadmill at low speed and elevation.

While the amount of weight being lifted is impressive, notice the way the weights are increased gradually and that rest between lifts increases as the weights increase. Yes, the final weight is extremely heavy, but Jason worked up to it gradually with adequate rest between lifts.

Day 2 involves five different exercises, which are less on weights and more on reps, done in sequence, and which Jason calls the Big Five 55 Workout. He alternates between five exercises: front squats, pull-ups, push-ups, power clean lifts (bend down, lift the barbell to the chest, hold erect, then lower), and hanging on the pull-up bar while pulling knees up to elbows. He does 10 sets, with minimal rest in between that eventually total 55 reps for each of the five exercises.

Statham alternates between the five exercises and performs the entire circuit 10 times. He starts with 10 reps, then goes down to nine, then eight, and so on, making for a total of 55 reps per exercise. There should be minimal rest time between each set.

Day 3, for a change of pace, is mostly aerobic done entirely on the rowing machine. He warms up slowly on the machine for 10 minutes, then performs six high-intensity sprints, each covering 500 meters, in one minute, 40 seconds average time, which is very fast. He cools down by walking 500 meters carrying two heavy kettle weights.

Daniel Craig

The most rugged and muscular of the actors to star in the *James Bond movies*, Daniel Craig looks like he can handle any situation or antagonist. His workouts have built a physique that looks powerful, yet functional, with flexibility and speed as well as considerable strength. What is his workout like?

He starts the week performing a power circuit that works the full body, not just one or two muscle groups, and performs three sets of 10 reps. This series includes exercises for the arms and shoulders, chest, abdominals and center body core, upper and lower back, and the legs, including glutes, quadriceps, hamstrings, and calves. For the next four days, Daniel exercises limited muscle groups, performing four sets of 10 reps. Every session concludes with a five-minute sprints interval on the treadmill or outside the fitness center. His trainer then has him take off from the gym for the weekend, but he has Daniel do some light yoga-style stretching and easy aerobic exercises, usually a swim or a run at a slow or moderate pace.

Day 2 workout. For example, the muscle group that Daniel exercises on Day 2 works the chest, shoulders, and back. The workout includes these four exercises, which you can try because they involve moderately heavy weights performed for 10 reps each:

1. **Incline barbell bench press**. The starting position is lying back on a bench raised to an incline. The barbell is raised to shoulder height with the palms facing forward. Exhale fully and press up the barbell with both arms. Hold in the fully extended position, then inhale before slowly returning to the starting position. Daniel performs four sets of 10 reps, with 90-second rests between sets.

2. **Pull-ups** are a bodyweight calisthenic exercise and begin by reaching up to grasp the pull-up bar or handles with palms facing forward and hands about shoulder-width apart. Slowly pull up to bring the chin to the level of the bar or handles, then slowly lower fully to the starting position. Squeeze your shoulder blades as you lift and exhale. Inhale as you lower back down. Again, perform four sets of 10 reps, with 90-second rests between sets.

3. **Incline press-ups** are a modified version of the classic push-up, and they are a little easier since you are not lowering all the way down and lifting up from the floor position. Place your hands shoulder-width apart on a bench and extend your legs fully to the rear. You should be up on your toes. Begin with your arms fully extended and slowly lower your chest to the bench, exhaling as you descend. Pause momentarily, and then raise fully back up to the starting position, inhaling as you rise. Perform four sets of 10 reps with 90-second rests between sets.

4. **Dumbbell incline fly** begins by lying on an incline bench and holding a dumbbell in each hand. Begin with arms fully extended upward. Slowly lower your arms outwards to the side until your arms are parallel to the floor or as far as you can comfortably lower without pain. It may be easier to have a slight bend at the elbow. Bring your arms up above you again, then repeat the movement. As with the other exercises in this group, perform four sets of 10 reps with 90- second rests between sets.

On other days, Daniel Craig performs a series of leg-strengthening exercises, and bicep curls and dips for arms and shoulders. Then, the weekend and no weights, but then on Monday, it's back to the full-body workout after the two days of rest.

Dwayne "The Rock" Johnson

The Rock needs no introduction, having gone from college athlete to WWE sensation to action movie star. Unlike many other Hollywood stars who are well built, Dwayne may be the best-built, most muscular star ever with the possible exception of Arnold Schwarzenegger. Dwayne makes it clear he worked hard to get where he is and to achieve his huge muscles, but he is always open to share his experience and practices to benefit others. While it is doubtful that any of us aspire to build up the muscle bulk he showed us in *Fast Five* or *Hercules* or to be anywhere near Dwayne's level, there may be value in letting him share his advice. He is inspiring, there's no doubt of that.

He starts with cardio. First thing in the morning every morning, The Rock hits the elliptical cross-training machine for 30 to 50 minutes of hard aerobics.

Then breakfast. He begins his day's fueling with a protein-intense breakfast. For example, on most days he consumes five serious meals, and the first one, after the early cardio and a shower, includes no less than:

➤ Two cups of cooked oatmeal (starts with one cup of dry oats)
➤ Three egg whites plus one whole egg (egg whites are almost pure protein)
➤ 10-ounce steak or other lean meat (for extra protein)

➤ One glass watermelon juice

The remaining four or so meals of the day each include an eight-ounce serving of either fish, chicken, or beef, along with vegetables. like broccoli, asparagus, and potato, plus lots of eggs and egg whites. The last meal is limited to 10 egg whites and casein protein.

The workout begins later in the morning. The Rock makes it as tough and as intense as he can to follow his philosophy of "epic pain, epic gain." This is not a workout discipline that you will want to emulate, but what Dwayne goes through to achieve his massive muscles and sharp definition gives you an idea of what the human body is capable of building. A small fraction of these muscles can still be impressive.

He works out six days a week and varies the routine from day to day to rest different muscle groups and for variety to prevent boredom.

Day 1 focuses on the legs. Note the moderate to high level of reps.	**Day 2** is devoted to back and shoulder muscles.
Barbell Squat: 4 sets of 12 reps	Pull-Ups: 3 sets to failure
Thigh Abductor: 4 sets of 12 reps	Bent-Over Barbell Row: 4 sets of 12 reps
Hack Squat: 4 sets of 12 reps	Wide-Grip Lat Pulldown: 4 sets of 12 reps
Leg Press: 4 sets of 25 reps	Bent-Over Barbell Row: 4 sets of 12 reps
Leg Extensions: 3 sets of 20 reps	One-Arm Dumbbell Row: 4 sets of 12 reps
Single-Leg Hack Squat: 4 sets of 12 reps	Barbell Deadlift: 3 sets of 10 reps
Romanian Deadlift: 4 sets of 10 reps	Inverted Row: 3 sets, to failure
Barbell Walking Lunge: 4 sets of 25 reps	Dumbbell Shrug: 4 sets of 12 reps
Seated Leg Curl: 3 sets of 20 reps	Back Hyperextensions: 4 sets of 12 reps

The week continues with Day 3 for the shoulders, Day 4 for arms and abs, Day 5 for the legs again, and Day 6 for the chest. Day 7 is a rest day with no workouts, and The Rock is reported to indulge in ice cream on this one day a week. Well deserved, it seems.

Hugh Jackman

During the 17 years he played Wolverine, a mutant with the steel knife-blade hands, in the *X-Men* movies, Hugh Jackman has been bulking up well-defined muscles by following a tough workout routine and a high-protein diet. His career has extended beyond action hero to a lead role in the musical *Les Miserables*.

A balanced diet. Yes, extra protein has been an essential part of Hugh's diet, but he is not a protein-obsessed fanatic. He balances his diet with healthy, unprocessed carbohydrates, including vegetables like sweet potatoes, broccoli, spinach, and avocado, which is credited with omega-3 antioxidants, plus niacin, beta-carotene, riboflavin, folate, magnesium, potassium, pantothenic acid, and vitamins. Carbs plus protein also come from whole grains, notably oatmeal and brown rice, which are high in antioxidants, vitamins, minerals, and digestion-benefiting fiber. Oats are also believed to lower LDL (bad) cholesterol.

Protein sources include eggs, fish for omega-3 fats, chicken, and lean beef. All in all, it's a protein-rich version of the Mediterranean diet, although there's no indication he also includes nuts, seeds, and beans in his diet.

Bulk and cut muscle. Hugh's trainer introduced him to a dual strategy workout routine with one type focusing on building muscle mass and the other aiming to provide more definition. Low-intensity/high-intensity intervals were included to emphasize lean muscle and minimize body fat.

Hugh's training has followed *progressive overload*, which is gradually increasing the weight being pulled, pushed, and lifted during each workout to ensure continual increases in strength. During a four-week cycle, the weight was increased for each of the first three weeks, then reduced for the fourth week with a corresponding increase in the number of reps.

The exercises that Hugh performed included barbell bench press, back squat, weighted pull-up, and barbell deadlift, according to this four-week plan with progressions during the first three weeks:

Hugh Jackman's four-week progressive overload schedule:

Week 1:	Week 2:
5 reps at 60% of maximum in set one	4 reps at 65% of maximum in set one
5 reps at 65% of maximum in set two	4 reps at 75% of maximum in set two
5 reps at 70% of maximum in set three	4 reps at 85% of maximum in set three
5 reps at 75% of maximum in set four	4 reps at 85% of maximum in set four
Week 3:	**Week 4:**
3 reps at 70% of maximum in set one	10 reps at 40% of maximum in set one
3 reps at 80% of maximum in set two	10 reps at 50% of maximum in set two
3 reps at 90% of maximum in set three	10 reps at 60% of maximum in set three
3 reps at 90% of maximum in set four	10 reps at 90% of maximum in set four

Interestingly, Hugh's trainer concentrated his workout with only five major exercises to build arms and shoulders, chest, abs, back, and legs.

Now, with your motivation to build muscles and begin a successful weightlifting and fitness program, it's time to move on to your action plan in Chapter 4.

Chapter 4:

Optimal Exercise Routines and Recovery

Practices

With the lessons and insights we've now covered, and with an understanding of why heavy weights have the advantage over lighter weights, you are ready to develop your own exercise selection and recovery routine. This chapter is where you will learn the exercise routines that you can select to develop a personalized, effective schedule of workouts. While you will be doing many of your exercises with heavy weights, they may not be as heavy as the weights you lifted when you were younger (if you ever lifted weights during that time of your life) or that you may see others lifting.

Weightlifting is not limited to iron weights and machines with cables. It also includes bodyweight calisthenics, movements that require only the weight of your body to provide the necessary resistance for tough workouts that lead to impressive results.

To supplement calisthenics, those working out at home without equipment can purchase stretch bands or tubes that can be used to replicate many of the exercises performed at fitness centers with weights and progressive resistance machines. The exercises presented in this chapter will be weightlifting with weights and bodyweight calisthenics.

Most weightlifting exercises can be performed without risk at age 40-plus as long as you work progressively and don't try to lift too much. Stay fully aware of the necessary recovery time after weightlifting to let hypertrophy, the rebuilding and growth process, function and be cognizant that after age 40, hypertrophy takes longer and the risk of injury from overwork is greater. As you were advised in this book's introduction, patience will be rewarded with results; it takes time as well as effort to build lean, well-defined muscles.

The Right Routine for Your Age

Your age, like most numerical designations, is relative. At age 40, or 50, or 60, your ability to perform a range of weightlifting exercises with varying weights and reps depends on your current physical state.

Your condition is based on a diversity of factors, including how aging has affected you, like the degrees of joint and tendon flexibility, and how they may have stiffened; how your health is; whether your muscles have atrophied from lack of use; and whether your cardiovascular system is running at full functionality. As it has been said, "It's not the years, it's the miles," meaning your condition is not just about age, but what damage has occurred from under-use or over-use. It is important to treat your body with respect for its actual condition and not what you hope or wish it to be. Realism is important if you are to achieve your expectations of greater strength, bigger muscles, and overall fitness.

First, Do No Harm

Yes, you will be working hard and challenging your muscles, joints, tendons, and ligaments, but your objective is to build and grow, not to punish and injure.

Whatever your condition now, respect your body as being middle-aged and follow the Hippocratic doctrine of "first, do no harm." You may have the best of intentions, but if you start out doing exercises that are best left to experienced, well-conditioned athletes or try to lift more weight than your joints or ligaments can handle, you are taking several unnecessary risks:

➤ **Injury** from a torn shoulder rotator cuff to a strained muscle that holds your kneecap in place. These kinds of injuries can take months to heal. There is minimal risk of injury if you work within your zone of ability.

➤ **Overuse,** meaning the muscles have been overextended, and the damage done to the fibers and cells will not repair and recover during the normal two days of rest. As a result, muscles will not grow and may atrophy, or get smaller.

➤ **Pain,** since lifting or pulling too much weight or doing too many reps can hurt and could end up diminishing your enthusiasm and motivation for strength training. Always consider pain to be a warning.

Your age, physical condition, health, and other factors make you unique. This is why you are being counseled to pay no attention to other weightlifters. They have their limits, and you have yours. There is no value in over-lifting, in pushing or pulling too much early in your middle-age return to weightlifting, only to injure yourself with a strained or torn muscle and shut down what you have just started.

Exercises to Avoid in Middle-Age

Aside from lifting too much weight, there are popular exercises you may be familiar with and plan to include in your routine, but experts advise you to let these go and avoid the risks of injury. Tell yourself that you have outgrown these exercises and leave them to the youngsters:

➤ **Overhead press.** Standing and raising a barbell above your head and lowering to your shoulders behind your head puts excess pressure on your shoulders, neck, and spine.

➤ **Bench press.** Lying on a bench and pushing a heavy barbell upwards may be good for your chest at age 25, but at 45, an excess strain is put on your pectoral (chest) muscles, wrists, and shoulders.

➤ **Crunches.** These slight lifts of the head and shoulders while on your back replaced the sit-up as safer, but at middle age, crunches put too much pressure on your neck and spine. Avoid pinched nerves and work your abs with less risk by doing leg raises, hanging leg raises, and planks.

➤ **Deadlifts.** Bending down and lifting a barbell to your chest is dangerous to your back. As a minimum, deadlifts can cause chronic back pain and may result in more serious back injuries.

➤ **Leg presses.** Sitting and pushing a heavy weight with your legs bent seems innocent enough, but the pressure on middle-aged hips and knees can lead to joint pain. Instead, strengthen your legs with low-impact lunges while carrying a moderate weight dumbbell or no added weight.

➤ **Lateral pull-downs.** You sit on a bench, facing the machine, reach up and pull down a bar to your chest, or worse, behind your neck. At middle-age, this maneuver risks pinched neck nerves and torn rotator-cuff shoulder muscles.

Also, while you are encouraged to include cardiovascular training into your workouts, be aware that running on hard surfaces can cause permanent knee damage, and you should consider limiting running to a treadmill or on grass if you want to run outdoors. Runners need to wear quality shoes designed for cushioned landing and to help prevent pronation, or outward foot rotation.

Equipment You Will Need (and Alternatives)

Fitness centers. The practice of strength training requires forms of resistance that are the basis of building lean, defined muscle, and making you stronger. There is usually a full range of weightlifting equipment found in a health club or fitness center, such as free weights like dumbbells, barbells, and kettlebells, plus progressive exercise machines with cables and weights that you can pull or push to work different muscle groups. A well-equipped fitness center or gym will also have rubber stretch tubes, adjustable benches, and a pull-up bar. These fitness centers generally require monthly membership fees unless you live in an apartment building or residential community that provides a fitness center as an amenity.

Home gym. A good alternative to a health club membership is to create your own small home gym, which could include a selection of free weights, a portable pull-up and chin-up bar, and a selection of stretchable rubber bands or tubes. The small investment in this equipment may be quickly amortized by the savings in fitness center monthly membership fees.

Bodyweight calisthenics. An even less costly way to build muscles and strength is to use your own weight as the resistance. Examples include familiar push-ups, pull-ups and chin-ups, leg raises, planks, and dips. There are many other calisthenics movements that can round out a full, total-body workout.

Group 1 of weightlifting exercises is based on having access to weights and other resistance equipment. **Group 2,** calisthenics, is almost all equipment-free and can be performed at home. You are encouraged to try exercises from both groups to add variety to your workouts and give a wider range of challenges to your muscles.

Each exercise has images of the movement and a link to a YouTube video demonstration so you can learn the movements correctly.

➤ **Skip Ad.** Many of the videos will begin with a short commercial, but after five seconds a "Skip Ad" box will appear on the lower right corner of the screen, and a quick click will get the exercise demo going.

Group 1: Weightlifting Exercises

The following weightlifting exercises have been selected to provide good strength and muscle building results with a low risk of injury. Select exercises to work specific muscle groups, and then vary them so you have at least one, preferably two, rest days before working the same muscle groups.

> ➤ **Tip:** Breathe out as you lift, and inhale as the weights are lowered.

> ➤ **Tip:** The weight you select should be what you can lift eight to 10 reps, and you should perform three sets with 60 to 90 seconds rest between sets.

1. Dumbbell Incline Press

You will develop your chest, upper arms, shoulders, and lats (sides of the upper chest) with the dumbbell incline press.

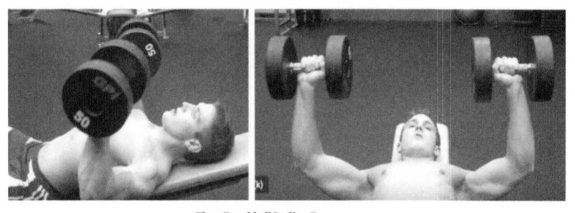

Fig 1. Dumbbell Incline Press

Tip: Use a lighter weight than you think appropriate when you perform the dumbbell incline press for the first few times. You do not want to over-lift or be trying to control the dumbbells because they are too heavy.

Tip: If the dumbbells are still hard to control, try the movement with a barbell. Use a wide grip (just past shoulder width) to simulate the movement with barbells.

Link to demonstration video: "How to: dumbbell incline chest press." *YouTube.* https://www.youtube.com/watch?v=8iPEnn-ltC8

2. Seated Cable Rows

This is a compound exercise that builds up the shoulders, abdominals, and core, both front and back.

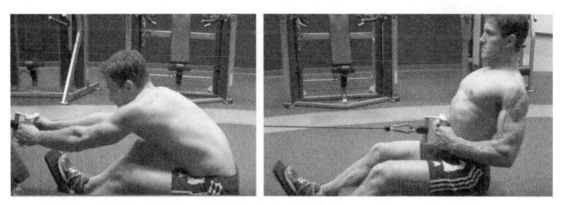

Fig 2. Seated Cable Rows

Tip: This is an excellent exercise for the hard-to-reach back muscles, but be careful to pull a weight you can manage without straining your back.

Tip: As you reach the full extend of the pull-back, squeeze your shoulder blades together for additional conditioning.

Link to demonstration video: "How to: seated low row." *YouTube.* https://www.youtube.com/watch?v=GZbfZ033f74

3. Dumbbell Split Squats

This leg exercise specifically works the quadriceps, the major muscles at the front of your thighs.

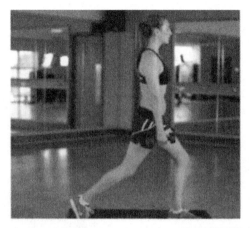 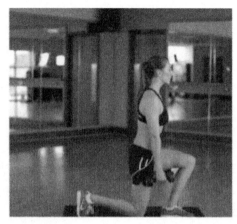

Fig 3. Dumbbell Split Squats

➤ **Tip:** Do not lean backward to maintain balance and keep control of the movement, but a slight forward lean is OK.

➤ **Tip:** Perform eight to 10 repetitions with the same leg forward, then switch to the other leg, and repeat to complete one set, remembering to keep your weight on the lead foot.

➤ **Tip:** If you find doing eight reps with each leg too difficult, use lighter dumbbells and few reps for the first week; do three sets with a rest of 90 seconds between sets.

Link to demonstration video: "Dumbbell split squat - fitness gym training." *YouTube.* https://www.youtube.com/watch?v=MEG6blZtUpc

4. Bent-Over Rows with Dumbbells

This will isolate the muscles in your back, especially the rhomboids, lats, and trapezoids. Secondarily you will be working the upper arm biceps and posterior deltoids, and you will also help stabilize your core and lower body.

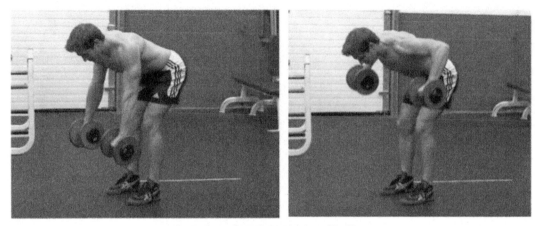

Fig. 4. Bent Over Rows with Dumbbells

➤ **Tip:** If you feel your back straining, reduce the amount of the forward bend, which will take some pressure off your spine.

➤ **Tip:** An alternative grip is to hold the dumbbells with your palms facing to the rear. (You can alternate grip with palms to sides and palms to rear between reps or sets; this will increase the muscles involved.)

Link to demonstration video: "How to: dumbbell bent-over row." *YouTube.* https://www.youtube.com/watch?v=6TSP1TRMUzs

5. Dumbbell Upright Row

This is a good shoulder-strengthening exercise and has considerable benefits when performed correctly. However, trainers caution that if performed incorrectly, upright rows can do more harm than good, so pay close attention to your form. Start with lighter weights to play it safe when starting out.

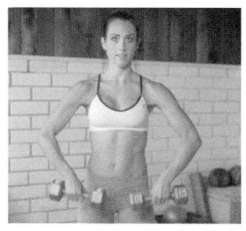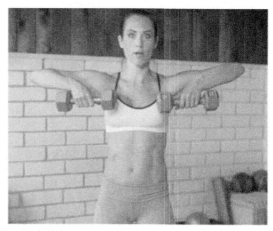

Fig 5. Dumbbell Upright Row

➤ **Tip:** Since you will be starting with lighter weights for safety, perform 12 to 14 reps for each of three sets with 60 seconds rest between sets. If you can't do 12 reps, reduce the weight you are lifting.

Link to demonstration video: "How to upright row - proper form and tips." *YouTube.* https://www.youtube.com/watch?v=VIoihl5ZZzM

6. Standing Barbell Curl

This is an exercise that weightlifters favor to build their upper arms, notably the biceps. It may also be performed with two dumbbells, but a barbell is preferred when starting out because it's easier to control and will tend to follow the correct path of up-and-down movements.

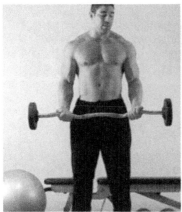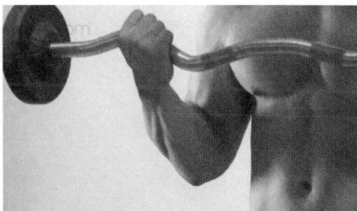

Fig 6. Standing Barbell Curl

> ➤ **Tip:** Be careful to control the bar, lifting it with both of your arms doing equal work (which will keep the bar parallel to the floor), and do not jerk the weight upwards, or let it drop down too fast. As with all weightlifting, slower is better.

> ➤ **Tip:** If you are able, perform three sets of eight to 10 reps with a rest of 60 to 90 seconds between sets. If you find doing eight reps too difficult, use a lighter barbell.

Link to demonstration video: "How to do a barbell curl | arm workout." *Howcast/YouTube.* https://www.youtube.com/watch?v=kwG2ipFRgfo

7. Dumbbell Side Lateral Raises

These side raises are excellent for building your shoulders and giving you a wide upper body. It challenges your rear deltoids and trapezius, but it's important to perform the movements correctly because, as you know by now, the rotator cuff muscles in your shoulder can be susceptible to strains and tears.

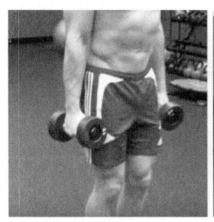 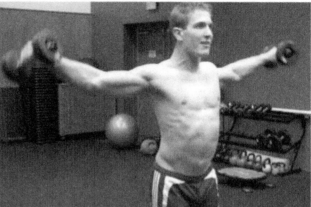

Fig 7. Dumbbell Side Lateral Raises

> ➤ **Tip:** If you feel pain, especially as you reach the top of the movement, stop and lower the weight. Be careful not to go any higher in the following reps (your range of motion should increase over time).

> ➤ **Tip:** Perform three sets of eight to 10 reps, with a rest of 60 to 75 seconds between sets. If you can't make it to eight reps in the first set, stop when you must, then reduce the weight for the next two sets.

Link to demonstration video: "How to: dumbbell lateral side raise." *YouTube.* https://www.youtube.com/watch?v=3VcKaXpzqRo

Group 2: Calisthenic Exercises

Bodyweight calisthenics can be performed at home, or anywhere, with little or no special equipment, and they should be part of your weightlifting program even if you have access to a fitness center's equipment. You may combine weightlifting and calisthenics in a single workout or on alternate days. Just be sure to avoid working the same muscle groups on consecutive days.

➤ **Tip:** For all exercises performed on the floor, use a yoga, exercise mat, or carpeting for cushioning. It's important to protect your spine.

➤ **Tip:** Breathe out as you lift or push yourself up, and inhale as your bodyweight is lowered.

➤ **Tip:** You can't vary your bodyweight, so for optimal effects, slow down the pace of the movements so you can lift or pull about 10 reps. For example, if you are finding it hard to do 10 push-ups, take a few seconds longer during each up and down.

➤ **Tip:** Perform three sets with 60 to 75 seconds rest between sets.

8. Planks

The plank looks simple enough, just holding a position, but it is a static stability exercise credited as outstanding for strengthening the core, which includes your abdominals, back, and sides. The plank is recommended as a replacement for sit-ups, which may cause spinal damage through disc compression.

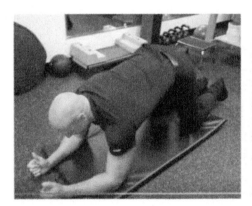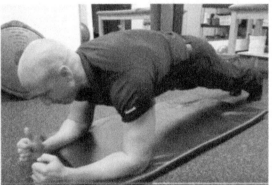

Fig 8. Planks

➤ **Tip:** Correct posture is critical. The objective is to keep your back straight, not sagging or with your buttocks pushing upward. Do not raise your head, but hold it so you are looking at the floor.

➤ **Tip:** This is the plank position, or pose, and it is held for 10 seconds up to one minute. One plank rep is considered one set, so you should perform three planks with a 60- to 90-second rest between planks.

➤ **Tip:** Within several weeks, you should be able to hold your plank, with a straight back, for 45 to 60 seconds.

Link to demonstration video: "How to do a proper plank." *Body Mind Wellness Clinic/YouTube.* https://www.youtube.com/watch?v=gvHVdNVBu6s

9. Bodyweight Squats

This is a classic bodyweight exercise that is an excellent builder for the quadriceps and hip flexors.

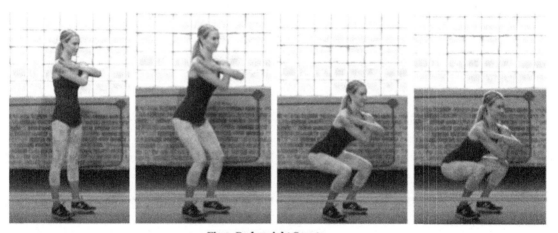

Fig 9. Bodyweight Squats

➤ **Tip:** If you find doing eight reps too difficult, perform fewer reps for the first week or two until your legs are accustomed to the movement.

➤ **Tip:** If your knees hurt during, or following, the squats, limit your descent to just before your thighs are parallel with the floor, but not past the point when the knee pain begins.

Link to demonstration video: "How to do a body-weight squat." *Health Magazine/YouTube.* https://www.youtube.com/watch?v=LyidZ42Iy9Q

10. Lying Leg Raises

Leg raises, like the plank, can replace sit-ups and crunches (partial sit-ups) to work the abdominals and core. This movement also stretches the hip flexors, hamstrings, and glutes.

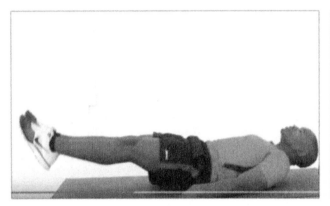 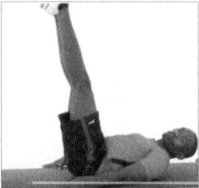

Fig 10. Lying Leg Raises

➤ **Tip:** You may find it easier to raise your legs if you slide your hands under your hips; alternatively, place a folded towel under your hips. This may also prevent straining your lower back muscles.

Link to demonstration video: "How to do lying leg raises for abs." *YouTube.* https://www.youtube.com/watch?v=UvcTNVbjTYo

11. Push-Ups

This is a classic bodyweight exercise that has stood the test of time, being safe to perform, and returning good results in strengthening many muscle groups, including arms, shoulders, back, abdominals, and core.

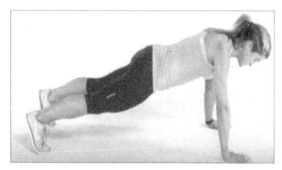 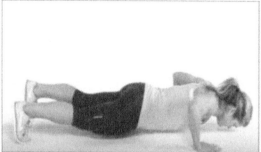

Fig 11. Push Ups

➤ **Tip:** As you get stronger, and push-ups get easier, slow down each cycle, taking longer to go down and back up. This can challenge your muscles more than simply increasing the reps.

➤ **Tip:** If you are having trouble doing even one or two push-ups, begin by keeping your weight on your knees instead of your toes. Or, place your hands on a bench, so you are not fully lowering to the floor.

Link to demonstration video: "How to do a push-up." *Dr. Oz/YouTube.*
https://www.youtube.com/watch?v=rjc0O7OXS3g

12. Pull-Ups and Chin-Ups

Pull-ups and chin-ups will build your upper back, shoulders, and core; chin-ups also give your biceps good resistance. You may have done pull-ups in high school, and if you thought they were tough then, wait until you try them now at middle-age. But you can work your way back and get quite good at pull-ups.

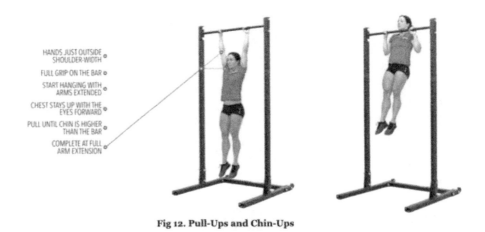

HANDS JUST OUTSIDE SHOULDER-WIDTH

FULL GRIP ON THE BAR

START HANGING WITH ARMS EXTENDED

CHEST STAYS UP WITH THE EYES FORWARD

PULL UNTIL CHIN IS HIGHER THAN THE BAR

COMPLETE AT FULL ARM EXTENSION

Fig 12. Pull-Ups and Chin-Ups

➤ **Tip:** You may alternate pull-ups and chin-ups. For example, set one, pull-ups; set two, chin-ups; and set three, return to pull-ups. The only difference is the grip (palms forward, wide grip for pull-ups; palms back, narrow grip for chin-ups).

➤ **Tip:** Repeat the cycle until you have performed five to eight reps. If you can only do one or two reps, that's OK; it's better to do fewer pull-ups in the correct form than to do more by lifting partially, or going too fast.)

Link to demonstration video: "The strict pull-up and chin-up." *YouTube.* https://www.youtube.com/watch?v=HRV5YKKaeVw

13. Hanging Leg Lifts

This exercise is another good challenge to the core muscles, especially your abdominals, back, and shoulders. It requires a pull-up bar and can be approached in three gradual stages. You are free to go directly to Stage 3, but it's a good idea to make sure you can perform Stages 1 and 2 before trying Stage 3.

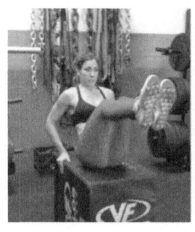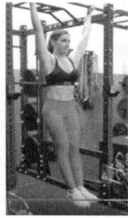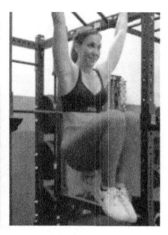

Fig 13. Hanging Leg Lifts

➤ **Tip:** In the early stages of your fitness program, you may find hanging from the bar difficult. In time you will get stronger, but if necessary, practice the first two stages (as shown in the video demo).

➤ **Tip:** In the interim, before you can perform this exercise, rely on lying leg raises and planks to tighten your core muscles.

Link to demonstration video: "Hanging leg raises done right." *YouTube.* https://www.youtube.com/watch?v=lS5B0MmLgZs

14. Triceps Bench Dips

This simple exercise can be performed using a bench, low table, or chair, and it is one of the best movements to isolate and work the triceps muscles at the rear of your upper arms. If you use a chair, make sure it is solid and will not tip forward as you place your weight on it.

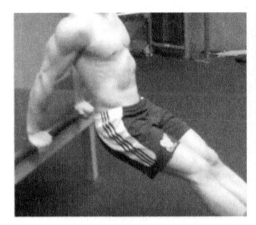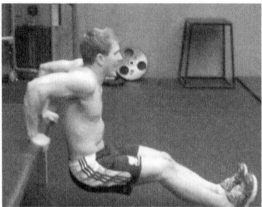

Fig 14. Triceps Bench Dips

➤ **Tip:** If this exercise is too difficult, bring your feet back so they are closer to the chair or bench, for example, so your feet are just two feet in front. Or, only lower yourself partially during the descent.

Link to demonstration video: "How to: triceps bench dips. *YouTube.* https://www.youtube.com/watch?v=c3ZGl4pAwZ4

Remember Rest and Recovery

At the risk of being repetitive, this is a reminder to give rest and recovery time their correct amount of attention if you want to optimize the results of your weightlifting and strengthening efforts. It can be tempting, especially when you are just getting started, to be enthusiastic and want to give it your all. It can be hard *not to workout!*

But, as you know by now, hypertrophy, the biological process that you will depend on to build muscles, is based on proteins and their component amino acids repairing and rebuilding the muscle cells and fibers damaged during lifting weights. Hypertrophy can only be functional when the muscles are allowed to rest for one or two days. At age 40-plus, two days is the preferable recovery time, and three days is even better.

Can You Lift Weights Every Day?

The answer to that question is both no and yes; it's a function of which muscles are being exercised on consecutive days:

> ➤ **No,** you should not exercise the same muscles or muscle groups on consecutive days. If you do chin-ups and barbell curls on Monday, your biceps and shoulders will not appreciate another round on Tuesday. The damage done to the muscles will not repair or grow to achieve over-rebuilding. Over time, what is medically called *repeated insults* will shrink the muscles and leave them weaker rather than stronger.

> ➤ **Yes,** if you work different muscles and muscle groups and allow the necessary rest time between workouts of the same muscles. For example, you could do the biceps and shoulders work on Monday, leg raises and squats on Tuesday, and then planks and seated cable rows on Wednesday, giving the biceps two full days to recover.

Can You Work Your Total Body?

While many weightlifters prefer shorter sessions, concentrating on a selective group of muscles, and getting their workouts done on five, six, or seven days each week, others prefer the alternative of working everything hard during one session, performing a complete routine of full-body exercises in a single workout session. During 40 or 50 minutes, they cover the arms and shoulders, chest and upper body, core, including the abdominals, back, upper and lower legs. So, the question is, can you, in middle-age, do this safely and productively?

> ➤ **Yes,** if it is done correctly and the need for rest and recovery is respected. You need to take two days of rest (or three) before repeating the full-body routine.

> ➤ Be aware that a total-body weightlifting workout takes longer than if you are concentrating on just two or three muscle groups. It can also be more of an exertion and can leave less experienced weightlifters exhausted.

➤ An advantage of fewer weightlifting sessions per week is that it leaves more days open for cardiovascular workouts. If you have allocated 40 or 45 minutes per day to work out, you can dedicate most of that time to running, fast walking, swimming, cycling, or hitting the elliptical and stair-climbing machines.

➤ Be sure to do light stretching before working out and then more stretching after the workout. We'll cover stretching in the next chapter.

When to Consult Your Doctor

In the spirit of "do no harm," as a middle-aged person who is beginning an exercise routine (or returning after a long layoff), it is important to take care of yourself and avoid injury. So should you see a doctor before beginning your workouts, or if you are experiencing pain or discomfort during or after exercise? The answer is yes to both questions.

See Your Doctor (1)

At this age, you should be having an annual physical exam with all of your vital signs checked out. Your doctor may refer you to a specialist, such as a cardiologist, to check your heart health, or an orthopedist if there are any joint or bone issues of concern. It's far better to confront potential problems early. It is normal and common for persons of middle-age to have aches and pains with the normal wear and tear of a life lived actively.

Even if you feel great and have no history of heart disease, getting your heart condition evaluated makes sense. A blood test will give a reading on a range of bodily conditions, and in particular, your doctor will probably check your blood lipids, which include HDL (good), LDL (bad) cholesterol, and triglycerides, and may even run an EKG to see your heart's electrical patterns. The doctor will listen carefully to your heartbeat and how your breathing is doing. A nurse will check your weight and blood pressure.

If you head to the cardiologist for a more in-depth analysis, you may take an exercise stress test to measure your heart's aerobic capacity or a CT scan to see how effectively your heart is pumping blood and if there are any arterial deposits. Rest assured that elevated levels of LDL cholesterol and triglycerides are easily treated today with inexpensive medications, notably statins, so don't put off getting checked out once you are age 40-plus. Hypertension (high blood pressure) is also potentially serious, yet treatable with a wide range of medications.

Your lifestyle should be evaluated, especially if you are overweight or obese, and the doctor may make dietary recommendations. (Chapter 6 will give you a good understanding of how to adopt a healthy diet.)

See Your Doctor (2)

There are many reasons that your workouts may prompt you to see your doctor, possibly having to do with heart-related concerns, or a joint, muscle, or tendon injury. Follow the warning that is posted on most aerobic exercise machines: if you feel pain in the chest, or become lightheaded, dizzy, or nauseous, stop and seek medical attention. It may be nothing, perhaps indigestion, or it may be a warning that something in your cardiovascular system needs prompt attention.

When the pain and discomfort in a joint are continuous and disruptive to normal activity, it is time to see the orthopedist, many of whom have training in sports medicine and are experienced with exercise-induced injuries. In many cases, you may be advised to follow the R.I.C.E. discipline: rest, ice, compression, and elevation. Certain joint injuries may require a cortisone injection to reduce inflammation and promote healing.

In summary, a little pain and discomfort is a normal result of lifting weights and working out. Use good sense when it comes to the amount of weight you are lifting, and be sure to respect the rest and recovery disciplines. Be alert to when the pain becomes serious, and do not ignore its warnings. The earlier that physical problems are diagnosed and treated, the faster the recovery.

Now, it's on to Chapter 5 with some more ideas about how to get your workouts going and keep them going.

Chapter 5:

Metabolism, Motivation, Commitment

The objective of this chapter is to help you to understand what will make the difference in your being able to achieve the goals you are imagining for yourself as an aspiring weightlifter and fitness enthusiast. You may have tried weightlifting and bodybuilding before but gave it up as other responsibilities began to compete for your time and attention. Your energy level began to diminish, and you found the weights becoming heavier rather than lighter. You may have been a runner at one time, but that drifted away, too.

Or, this could all be new to you. You never (or almost never) lifted weights or did serious bodyweight calisthenics. Cardiovascular conditioning? No time, no interest?

No matter, you're here now and ready to step up to the challenges and rewards of getting more lean muscle, getting stronger, and being in overall good, healthy condition. You may be excited about getting started on the weightlifting and bodyweight calisthenics in the previous chapter, and that's great. But first, take a little time to understand why things are different for you now at middle-age, and why that is.

Continuity in your workouts and attention to your diet are essential, and they are for a reason beyond the basics of working out hard, getting adequate rest, and seeing positive results. As you age, things are slowing down, and muscle mass is diminishing. Why?

Metabolism: The Unseen Factor

Do you wonder why a person like yourself, who is middle-aged, cannot build muscle tissue and achieve bulk like someone in his 20s? Why does someone in their 40s lose muscle mass at a faster rate than someone in their 20s? Why does fat tend to build up more quickly, and why do the pounds add up even though you are eating the same amount as when you were younger? Now that you're age 40, 50, or more, there is an unseen factor that you need to understand and manage. It's your metabolism, the sum total of your body's biological and chemical cellular processing. At your age, it's slower than it used to be, and your fitness and dietary programs need to be adjusted to reverse the decline of your current metabolic rate.

Losing Muscle Mass

Lifestyle factors contribute to the slowing of your metabolism. You may be aware that most middle-aged people tend to follow a less active, more sedentary lifestyle that contributes to muscle loss, and it makes your commitment to a serious physical fitness routine much more important. But also, apart from your behavior, it is natural for you to experience muscle loss and the aging of your metabolic system.

Age-related muscle loss is called sarcopenia, and it is a normal, natural part of growing older. According to *Harvard Health Publishing* (2016), after age 30, you can lose from 3 percent to 5 percent of your muscle mass each decade. Men lose more muscle than women; on average 30 percent of their muscle mass disappears throughout their lifetimes.

But this degree of muscle loss is not inevitable, and muscle mass can be increased, rather than decreased, with a commitment to a good weightlifting program of resistance exercises that continues throughout middle-age.

Lost muscle mass can be recovered, according to Dr. Thomas W. Storer, director of Brigham and Women's Hospital's physical function and exercise physiology laboratory. He says that it takes work, planning, and dedication, but "it is never too late to rebuild muscle and maintain it" (2016).

The muscle loss, sarcopenia, is traced to declines in testosterone, and studies have been conducted to determine if testosterone supplements can slow or reverse muscle mass loss. While some results were positive, there were adverse effects, and the FDA has not approved testosterone supplements for building muscle mass in men.

As a result, Dr. Storer concludes that the optimal approach to building lean muscle mass, regardless of your age, is a continuing program of progressive resistance training: gradually increasing your workout volume by raising the amount of weight being lifted, and maintaining the number of reps and sets as your strength and endurance improve.

Metabolic Consumption Rates

Your metabolic rate directly affects the number of calories you burn in a day. This rate of caloric consumption is expressed in several ways:

➤ Your **resting** metabolic rate is measured when you are asleep, immobile, and resting and is the lowest rate that can sustain basic reflexes that keep you alive, including energy consumption to maintain your heartbeat, breathing, and brain functions. You burn the least number of calories per hour when in the resting state

➤ The **thermic** effect of food is the caloric consumption required to support digestion of the food you eat and process in a given period, including chewing and swallowing, grinding and acidification in the stomach, and the assimilation of food in the small and large intestines as it is carried through the GI tract by the contractions of peristalsis.

➤ **Non-exercise thermogenesis** includes all calories you burn while standing, sitting, writing, reading, speaking, laughing, doing light housework, and everything else that involves any physical effort except for exercise and digestion.

➤ **Exercise consumption** is the number of calories you burn during and immediately after exercise. This includes all active exercise, from walking to gardening, lifting and carrying, showering, stair climbing, jogging and running fast, weightlifting, swimming, and cycling, among other exertions.

The number of calories that are burned by these four categories varies from person to person based on individual metabolic rates and other factors, such as the type, amount, and intensity of the exercises and movements performed. Your metabolic rate can be affected by your age and certain physical characteristics such as muscle mass, height, weight, genetics, and hormones.

We'll get into calories and weight loss in the next chapter, but it's important to understand that weight gain, weight maintenance, and weight loss are entirely determined by two factors: the number of calories that are consumed and assimilated, and the number of calories that are metabolized. Any excess calories that exceed your daily needs and are not burned are stored as fat.

Raising Your Metabolism

Let's consider your metabolic control options. Can you influence the rate that your metabolism burns calories, especially since your metabolic rate is gradually declining with age? Exercise and other physical activities can have immediate positive effects on your metabolism and can also have a secondary effect during rest and even sleep:

> ➤ You can influence **non-exercise** thermogenesis by being a less sedentary, more active person, throughout the day. Walk instead of ride, take the stairs instead of the elevator, do your own housework, and fit some yoga stretching into your day (or Tai chi or Pilates), Avoid sitting as you work by arranging your laptop or desktop computer keyboard at a height that lets you work in a standing position at least part of the time. Over an average day, becoming more active and less sedentary can consume an additional 200, 600, or more calories as well as keeping you more flexible and healthier overall.

> ➤ **Exercise thermogenesis** can be an even more productive way to burn extra calories. The amount and intensity of the exercises are directly related to the calories, so, for example, a 40-minute weightlifting session can burn 500 to 600 calories compared to 40 to 80 calories consumed during that same time while sitting and watching TV or holding a conversation. Similarly, two miles on the treadmill, either jogging or fast walking, can burn 200 to 220 calories in 20 to 30 minutes compared to 20 or so calories consumed while sitting.

> ➤ **Muscle gain:** Studies show that age-related metabolic slowdown is connected to the loss of muscle mass so that using weightlifting to build muscle mass will result in a greater overall metabolism rate even during the sleeping and resting phase, when the metabolic rate is at its slowest. A 10 percent increase in resting metabolism can result in several hundred incremental calories burned overnight with no exertion on your part!

The **most effective discipline** is to combine both of these practices: to be more active and less sedentary since this can increase your metabolism throughout the day; and to exercise with weightlifting and aerobics at least three days a week. You can't affect your metabolism based on how your body digests and absorbs foods, but adding more physical activity to your daily routine can turn up the caloric burn rate when you are taking it easy, even while sleeping.

Appetite effects: Here's a heads up to alert you to an effect on your weight that might surprise you It can cause you to gain more weight rather than losing or maintaining your current weight, despite your adoption of a weightlifting and aerobics program:

➤ While increasing your exercise regimen and daily rate of activity will burn more calories, it will probably also increase your appetite. This can lead to taking in more calories than you burn.

➤ Be careful not to snack excessively, and when you do snack or increase serving sizes at meals, emphasize lean protein, which will keep you feeling full longer (protein is slower to digest), and is beneficial to the muscle-building process of hypertrophy.

Motivation and Commitment

An important part of your long-term muscle and strength-building program is mental. Of course, it will be the weights, the reps, the sets, and the rests in between that will give you the lean muscle mass you want, but your state of mind will determine if you actually get started and if you will go the distance for the months and years of exercise it will take. Rome wasn't built in a day, and your impressive physique won't happen immediately.

The Motivation

In the initial chapter and at other points in this book, the importance of motivation was established as an incentive to getting your weightlifting and fitness program underway. No one can make you get into a regular, well-planned weightlifting program; you have to have the resolve and enthusiasm to take charge of your body, your health, and your appearance:

➤ If you have read this far, chances are good that you get it, "you're in."

➤ You imagine yourself lifting the barbells and dumbbells, doing the push-ups and pull-ups, the planks, the squats, and the splits.

➤ You feel committed to cardiovascular conditioning to help melt the extra pounds while you invest in your health and longevity.

➤ You feel better looking in the mirror in anticipation of the bigger, defined muscles you are going to build.

The Commitment

But will you have the determination and discipline to go the distance, to continue regularly with your bodybuilding and strengthening practices? Motivation is important at the beginning, but you need to have the discipline to stick to the routine even on days when you just don't have the drive, when you say, "I'll do it tomorrow."

You need to transcend the forces that hold you back, to break free of the constraints, and be committed no matter how tired or uninspired you are at that moment. Only then can you keep on track to meet your fitness and strengthening goals.

Commitment to succeed as a weightlifter, who builds muscle, who loses fat and excess weight, starts in the mind, which is the most effective and persuasive tool that will help you achieve your bodybuilding objectives. A positive attitude and the determination to work through the toughest movements will carry you through the worst of it with grit. Those who fail to make it, who give up, who quit, may be tough physically but don't have the mental toughness. Remember that your body will follow your mind.

Successful weightlifters at every level of training have developed positive thoughts to get themselves to the gym, to pick up the first weight of the session, to get through it with a full effort, no matter how tired or busy they were. You can adopt these thoughts, make them yours, let them carry you to the workout, and through the work, every time.

Positive Reinforcements

1. *I'll just do a half-workout today, take it easy.*

   This works when you're tired and helps to get you started. In almost every case, once you get started and warmed up, you get into the movements, do all the reps, and go all the way. It's a little psychological game that you can play on yourself, and somehow it continues to work time after time. As it has been said, "just showing up is 90 percent of success," so just get those workout shoes and shorts on, get to a machine or a weight, and start out slowly. You'll warm up and keep going.

2. *The solo mountain climber's focus and discipline.*

When you are heading up the side of Yosemite's El Capitan, climbing without ropes or tools, there is no looking up or down, no thinking about what's coming or how hard it will be. The same applies to weightlifting when the only thing that matters is what you need to do at that moment: focus on the now. Another advantage of being in the moment while working out is the clearing of your mind, in a meditative way, so that all distractions are ignored. You will be calmer, and by paying close attention, your form and posture will be better, and you will be less likely to cause an injury.

3. *The mirror, the scale, and the tape measure.*

The numbers don't lie, exaggerate, or try to please your ego. They are the reality that will testify to the depth and duration of your commitment to building your body, getting your weight where it belongs, and getting that gut flatter. Start with a benchmark set of measurements, and check in every week. Look at yourself in the mirror without criticism or disappointment and just take notice of how your pecs (chest muscles) and abdominals look: a little soft, a layer of fat. Same for the arms and legs. Weigh yourself before breakfast, and write down the number each week, or daily if you prefer. Same for the tape measurement. Over time, you will see and record progress, and that will help solidify your commitment to your long-term objectives.

Inspirational Quotes

1. *"Tough times don't last, but tough people do."* — Richard Shuller (2020).

This quote applies to all aspects of life but has found special appreciation among professional lifters who push to their absolute limits. But especially for you as you are beginning weightlifting and conditioning, there are times when it isn't fun, like that last pull-up or barbell curl. Your thighs may be burning after three sets of squats or splits, and that last set of dumbbell rows may have you breathing pretty hard. But every time the set is over, and the rest begins, the pain and burning feeling subsides, and the workout always ends with a feeling of work well done, a sense of satisfaction. You are tough and getting tougher.

2. *"To be a champion, you must act like a champion."* — Lou Ferrigno (2020).

Lou Ferrigno, a champion weightlifter who played the Incredible Hulk, contributed to this recommended mindset because he believes that strength comes from within. A championship attitude is attainable by all of us if we believe in ourselves and envision the well-muscled, well-defined body we are working to achieve. But it goes further: If you want to become a well-built bodybuilder, you need to work out like one. Positive thinking is essential to motivate and inspire you, but without hard work and the determination to give it your all, positive thinking is just a dream.

3. *"Don't wish it were easier. Wish you were better."* — Jim Rohn (2020).

The thought leads us to expect that the workout, the lifting and pulling, the squatting and dipping, needs to be intensive, to challenge us. That leads to the realization that if it's easy, it's not being done right. You need to work to challenge your muscles to the point that muscle cells and fibers are damaged and need to self-repair through hypertrophy. The attitude that will carry you from passive to proactive is the recognition that it's a simple formula: strength is directly proportional to the effort that is invested in each workout. Of course, a hard workout can be followed in two days by a less intensive workout to aid recovery, but then be sure to make the next workout more intensive. It will pay off in the long-term.

4. *"It never gets easier. You just get stronger."* — Unknown (2020).

The idea is to add weights progressively when you can handle more without reducing reps, sets, or rest intervals. For example, head over to the dumbbell rack, and pick up a heavy weight you can do just one rep of a bicep curl or at most two. Do you wish you could do more reps? Find the weight you can lift or curl for eight reps and have the patience and confidence to know that in a reasonable time, with discipline, you will advance gradually from the lighter weight to the heavier ones and beyond. Just follow the basic practice of lifting weights that max out at eight to 10 reps, do the three sets, and be sure to rest between sets and between workouts.

5. *"You have to be at your strongest when you're feeling at your weakest."* — Unknown (2020).

This inspiration encourages weightlifters and cardio athletes to reach deep inside for the strength that they know is there. Imagine that you are a runner who is training for a marathon or other long-distance competition. The only time you can train is early in the morning before work, even in the cold and dark of winter. You need to roll out of bed at 5:30 a.m., wash your face, put on your running shoes, head outside, hit the road, and run into a biting cold headwind. What does it feel like to go through this, day after day, for months? This is what inner strength is all about, and it illustrates, in the extreme, what someone chooses to do to reach an objective. You probably will not have to work out under such an extreme condition. You'll be indoors, warm, lifting weights you can manage, and working to a reasonable, yet difficult peak of effort. But think of that runner in the dark, cold, early morning, and let it carry you to a better effort each day.

6. *"Strength does not come from physical capacity. It comes from an indomitable will."* — Mahatma Gandhi (2020).

The courage and determination that the leader of India's independence showed in standing up peacefully to overwhelming forces testify to the importance of resolve and commitment. Your willpower is what can help you accomplish what others think you cannot achieve. To friends, associates, and family, you may be wasting your time, risking injury, and for what? "You can't build muscles at your age," and "It's too late for you," they may say. Are they right? The answer is up to you. You can build muscle, get leaner and stronger, improve your health, well-being, and longevity if you have the will, the resolve to commit to a continuing program of progressive weightlifting, and aerobic training.

7. *"There are two types of pains, one that hurts you and the other that changes you."* — Unknown (2020).

A weightlifter's perspective. Too much pain can be harmful, but when you need to perform one more rep and the barbell feels like it weighs a ton, the discomfort of the extra effort that you need now won't last, but your satisfaction will. Too much pain can be dangerous, leading to injury and dampening your motivation to keep up with the regimen. But there is always some discomfort when you are trying to reach your peak output, and that is what you can expect, and need, to endure. The pain or strain you feel on the eighth or ninth rep won't hurt you; you are lifting or pulling the correct weight for your ability at that moment. It's the pain you feel on a first or second rep that is telling you the weight is too heavy for you, indicating you risk injury if you continue. Work progressively, and you will progress.

8. *"Pain is temporary. Quitting lasts forever."* — Lance Armstrong (2020).

The American prolific winner of the Tour de France has endured cycling up the mountains of the Alps and Massif Central while competing against the best bicyclists in the world. It was his resolve, his commitment, that kept him in the leader's yellow jersey to win seven successive tours. While nothing you will have to endure will approach the ordeal of a professional racer or weightlifter, you can learn and be inspired by their example. The intensity of their training is almost unimaginable, and frankly, the damage they are doing to their bodies can have long-term consequences. Don't try to imitate them, but let their "no quitting" attitude remind you on tough days that you will forget the momentary pain, discomfort, or inconvenience, but you may be disappointed in yourself if you don't go the distance.

Can you come up with your own quotes for motivation and commitment to building muscles and strength? All said, it's you who needs to be inspired, and no one knows you as well as you do. What makes you excited, enthusiastic, energized?

Now, a change of subjects. In Chapter 6, let's head into the kitchen and get the facts on how to eat better, healthier, and more satisfyingly to achieve your bodybuilding and strength-building goals.

Chapter 6:

Eating Right (and Loving It)

Eating Right in Middle-Age

The quality and composition of your diet are the most underrated aspects of physical fitness. Many people feel they have done the best they can for their fitness and health by spending hours every week in the fitness center or home gym, and they believe that gives them license to head into the kitchen and eat all they want of whatever they want. This is not correct.

There is truth to the adage, "you are what you eat," since your body is only able to assimilate and metabolize what you feed it. As you will see, a good diet will reward you in many ways, from keeping you leaner and helping to build muscles to giving you the energy and endurance you need to get stronger and get more done. Can your diet help you live longer? Yes, because a healthy diet will slow or stop the onset of heart disease, obesity, diabetes, chronic autoimmune disorders, gastrointestinal diseases, and degenerative diseases like Alzheimer's.

Your Three Essential Macronutrients

Nutritionists classify macronutrients as the three major food groups we've discussed: carbohydrates, proteins, and fats. These are separate from the many micronutrients like vitamins and minerals. There have been descriptions of the macronutrients in previous pages, but for clarity, let's get the definitions stated here. They are called "macro" because they are the larger amounts of food we eat, the totality of the calories we ingest, digest, assimilate, and metabolize.

Lindsey Wohlford, a wellness dietician at the MD Anderson Cancer Center, sums it up as the cornerstones of your diet:

➢ "Macronutrients are the nutritive components of food that the body needs for energy and to maintain the body's structure and systems" (2020).

Energy, structure, systems: the roles the macronutrients play are clearly defined.

Carbohydrates are your body's primary fuel, giving your muscles and your central nervous system the energy for movement, especially when the muscles are being worked or performing the exercise. According to Lindsey Wohlford, at least 45 percent and up to 65 percent of your daily caloric input should be from carbohydrates, or "carbs." We get our carbs from grains and cereals, fruits and vegetables, and foods containing sugar and other sweeteners. There is a popular misconception that carbohydrates are not good for us, but in reality, if they are from healthy sources like whole grains, fruits, and vegetables, and nuts and seeds, those are the essential carbs your body needs to keep going. There are four calories in one gram of carbs.

Protein is needed to give your body its structure, from muscles, ligaments, tendons, and bones, to skin and hair, organs, and nerves, down to cell membranes, and blood plasma. All are made from protein. Proteins are part of hormonal, enzyme, and metabolic systems and regulate the balance between acids and bases in your body. The recommended daily allowance (RDA) is 0.8 grams per kilogram of bodyweight, or 0.36 grams per pound, so a person weighing 150 pounds should consume about 50 grams of protein per day. However, when you are weightlifting to build muscles, your daily protein intake should be 75 grams or more. There are four calories in one gram of protein.

➤ The sources of protein in your diet are covered in detail later in this chapter.

Fats and oils (oils are fats that are liquid at room temperature) are your body's concentrated energy reserve and are higher in calories than the other two macronutrients. There are nine calories in one gram of fats, making storage easier. Stored fats can be called upon for energy when carbs (stored in the muscles as glycogen) are running low or depleted. Apart from energy, fats play a continuing role in providing insulation, protecting and cushioning your organs, and in the absorption and transport of fat-soluble nutrients, like vitamins D and E. The RDA for your daily fat consumption is between 20 percent and 35 percent of all calories, and saturated fats should be no more than 10 percent. Fats from extra virgin olive oil, avocados, and vegetable oils from soybeans, sunflower, safflower, and corn are monounsaturated or polyunsaturated and are recommended to promote cardiovascular health.

The 70:30 Rule of Fitness and Weight Management

Is achieving a high level of physical fitness and keeping your weight down attributable to 70 percent diet and only 30 percent physical training? The idea that diet is more than twice as important as working out has been popular among trainers and athletes for some time, but there does not appear to be a scientific basis for this precise ratio, although it is heading in the right direction. There is *scientific evidence* to show there are limits to how much exercise alone can contribute to weight loss.

As reported in the *Guardian* (2016), while exercise is definitely important for your health and well-being, research indicates that physical activity alone will not necessarily consume extra calories:

➤ Leading to the conclusion that diet should be the primary tactic to achieve weight loss.

This is based on studies that show that our metabolic processes reach a plateau beyond which additional exercise, whether it's weightlifting, cardio or both, does not continue the same rate of energy expenditures. Beyond a certain point, the body makes adjustments to constrain, or limit, how many calories are burned in a given time.

For example, after a day that included a long, intensive weightlifting and cardio workout from which you burned 650 extra calories, your metabolism may slow down more than normal while you're resting and asleep so your net calorie loss for the day is only 150 to 250 calories. Other studies reported in *Current Biology* (2016), which involved humans and other primates, showed that those who performed extra physical activity did not burn substantially more calories in 24 hours than those who performed moderate activity, but both groups did burn more calories than sedentary individuals whose activity levels were low.

At City University of New York, Professor Herman Ponzer, who participated in the study, said, "Exercise is really important for your health," but went further to conclude:

➤ "What our work adds is that we also need to focus on diet, particularly when it comes to managing our weight and preventing or reversing unhealthy weight gain" (2016).

Diet plays a larger role in maintaining a healthy weight and providing the essential nutrients for building muscle, maintaining a healthy metabolism, managing weight, and keeping a strong immune system to keep out disease and the incursions of aging.

Your body's health and strength, as well as your energy and endurance, are dependent upon the fuel you ingest and the quality and types of foods you eat. As important as weightlifting is to building muscles, and you're becoming stronger and more fit, your diet is as influential, possibly more so. In recognizing that our diet plays a key role in building muscle and keeping off fat, we'll help you cut through all the dietary misinformation and get you pointed to a lifelong dietary practice rather than a series of fad diets that come and go. There are fundamentals of nutrition that you will learn to follow.

Calories In, Calories Out

It's called the CICO diet, but it's not really a diet; it's a basic law of science. It stands for Calories In, Calories Out, and it means that weight maintenance is based on digesting the same number of calories that you burn each day. There are 3,500 calories in one pound of bodyweight, so if you wanted to lose one pound per week, you would have to take in 500 fewer calories than you burn each day in each week. The amount you burn is based on your unique metabolic rate, your activity level, and what you have ingested since certain foods are digested more readily and more completely than others.

> ➤ As you have just read in the previous section, exercise alone will not burn as many calories as you'd think.
> ➤ The way to improve the ratio of CICO is to take in fewer calories.

A calorie is simply a unit of energy. There are four calories in one gram of carbohydrate, four calories in a gram of protein, but nine calories in a gram of fat, which is nature's efficient way of storing energy and why foods that are high in fats and oils are, well, fattening.

Satiety: Feeling Full

One of the ways certain foods can be less or more fattening is their satiety level. The amount of fullness you feel slows how hungry you become and want to eat again. In general, foods that are high in protein are better at keeping you full longer because the complex protein molecules are harder for your digestive system to break down into their amino acid building blocks and then assimilate. This compares to the less complex molecules that compose carbohydrates and fats, which pass through the stomach and are digested much more quickly.

But even certain foods in the same categories have different satiety levels. A serving of boiled potatoes has the same number of calories from carbohydrates as a French pastry, like a croissant, but the potatoes are seven times more filling, research shows. This may be due to the carbohydrates in potatoes being composed of complex starches, which are slow to break down, and the croissant being made from two highly refined carbohydrates: white flour and sugar. It also contains butter, which also digests quickly.

The refined ingredients in the croissant illustrate the concerns that nutritionists have with highly refined and processed foods. Writing in *Today* (2020), registered dietician Samantha Cassetty says that instead of focusing just on calories:

➤ "It's better to be aware of your calorie needs and to develop an understanding of how calories from various foods make you feel."

➤ Controlling your appetite "with filling foods that are also in line with your body's calorie needs is a good way to manage your weight and your hunger levels," she concludes.

Limiting Highly Processed Foods

Highly processed foods account for about 60 percent of the average American diet and are blamed for adding excess calories, sodium (salt), chemical additives (for preservation, flavor enhancement, and color), saturated fats, and refined sugar. In consequence, this type of diet leads to weight gain, elevated levels of LDL (bad) cholesterol, high blood pressure, and higher blood sugar levels.

A small scale study reported in *Cell Metabolism* (2019) dramatically demonstrates the differences between a diet of highly processed foods and one of whole, unprocessed foods. Twenty participants first spent two weeks eating a processed diet exclusively, followed by the natural, unprocessed, whole foods. Both diets were matched with equal quantities of carbohydrates, protein, fats and oils, and fiber. Importantly, during the study, the participants were allowed to eat as much or as little as they wanted.

At the end of the study, the findings included:

➤ On the processed diet, participants ate an average of 500 calories per day more than on the whole foods diet and gained two pounds.

➤ When the same people switched to the unprocessed whole foods diet, they lost two pounds.

➤ It was noted that during the processed diet phase, participants ate faster and ate more, suggesting that the processed foods were less filling and signals of satiation were slower to reach the brain.

➤ It is also possible that faster and excessive eating was encouraged by higher amounts of salt and flavor enhancements in processed foods.

Conclusions include the reality that extra calories, regardless of the source, lead to weight gain, and further, it is postulated that unrefined, unprocessed foods, especially grains, are slower to be digested and absorbed, possibly due to high fiber content, and also raise resting metabolism rates.

The Importance of Protein in Middle-Age

Our bodies need carbohydrates, protein, and fats, but as a middle-age weightlifter aspiring to build muscle mass, your need for protein is greater than normal because you need that protein to build muscle tissue and to enable hypertrophy to function effectively. Being older, that need for protein is even greater.

Protein has specific benefits that benefit all people, but especially when you are middle-aged and want to pursue a physically active lifestyle.

1. Weight loss through appetite and hunger control. As noted, protein is slower to digest than carbohydrates and fats. It takes longer for the stomach acids and enzymes to break it down, so it stays there longer. There are weight-regulating hormonal factors as well:

➤ Ghrelin is a hunger stimulant that is suppressed by protein. This may be the result of the protein digesting slowly, causing the stomach to send a signal to the brain to slow down the release of ghrelin as if to say, "full house, no room here."

➤ Protein also invites the release of YY peptide, which is a hunger suppressant. It makes you feel full and less likely to reach for something else to eat.

In a study among overweight women, the participants increased their protein intake from 15 percent to 30 percent, and on average they consumed 441 fewer calories per day. That could cause the loss of one pound every eight days. The quantity of protein needed to reach 30 percent of a 2,000-calorie-per-day diet is equal to 600 calories, or 150 grams.

2. Reduced late-night snacking is another result of the "feeling fuller longer" effect of slow-digesting protein and the ghrelin and YY peptide appetite suppression effects. A study among overweight men, in which protein intake was increased to 25 percent of total calories, showed late-night cravings were reduced by 60 percent and the desire to snack at night was lowered by 50 percent.

3. The building block of muscle. Muscle cells and fibers are constructed of protein, During hypertrophy, when the muscle cells and fibers are being repaired following the damage that occurs during a weightlifting workout, protein is the "brick and mortar" that is piled on and patched in. Insufficient protein in the diet will retard hypertrophy and can lead to muscle loss.

> ➤ As an aspiring **middle-age weightlifter,** you need to be aware that your need for protein is greater than for those who are a decade or two younger. Your repair mechanisms and metabolism are slower and need more "raw materials" to patch up the damaged protein within your muscles.

4. Bones need protein, too. With age comes bone porosity, leading to osteoporosis and the risk of broken bones. While we think of calcium as the key component of bones (it is), protein plays an important role in helping to reinforce the calcium so that the bones are harder and less porous. This refutes the misconception that protein makes bones more fragile by leaching away the calcium; it's simply not true.

5. Faster metabolism and fat-burning. Eating and the process of digestion burns calories and fat because work is being done and energy is being expended. This process is called the thermic effect of food, and it varies depending on the food being digested. Protein's thermic effect is four times greater than when carbohydrates or fats are being digested, so it boosts metabolism and burns more calories. In one study, the higher protein diet burned about 100 more calories, and in another study that compared a high-protein group with a low-protein group, the net caloric burn for the high protein group was 260 calories per day.

6. Helps protect against heart disease. Analysis of 40 different studies of increased protein in the diet found that systolic blood pressure (top number) was lowered by 1.76 mm Hg, and diastolic pressure (bottom, smaller number) was lowered by 1.15 mm Hg. There was also a lowering of LDL (bad) cholesterol and triglycerides. These findings suggest a higher protein diet can help prevent strokes, heart attacks, and chronic kidney diseases.

7. Speeds recovery after injury. When you are injured, most of the damage is done to your skeletal muscles, which are made of protein, and those muscles need protein to repair themselves. Bone damage needs protein to speed repairs. A higher protein diet also increases platelets in the blood, which are used to clot and stop bleeding.

8. Maintaining your fitness as you age. A natural consequence of aging is the weakening of your muscles and reduction in muscle mass. The combination of increased protein in the diet and resistance exercises has been confirmed to prevent the onset of sarcopenia, which is age-induced muscle loss and deterioration. The exercise will encourage rebuilding and muscle growth, but adequate amounts of protein need to be available to allow hypertrophy to operate effectively.

Sources of Protein

The following are excellent sources of protein with additional muscle-building and health benefits. We begin with dairy and egg protein sources, then fish and seafood, then meat and plant sources.

Dairy and Egg Protein Sources

Greek yogurt is higher in protein than regular yogurt because it is strained to remove some of the water, thus concentrating what is left. There are 16 to 19 grams of protein in a ¾-cup serving, which is double that of regular yogurt. The protein in Greek yogurt is a combination of fast-digesting whey protein and slow-digesting casein protein. There is further benefit from the live probiotic bacteria cultures, which support the microbiome in the gut. Greek-style, high-protein yogurt is also available as Icelandic or Australian yogurt. Check the labels to be sure about the protein content. Choose low-fat or fat-free versions to save on calories and avoid saturated fats.

Milk is a good source of protein and carbohydrates, and while it can contain up to 4 percent partially saturated fats, there are low-fat and fat-free versions that are abundantly available (and recommended vs. full fat). The protein in milk, as in yogurt, contains both fast- and slow-digesting proteins, which are thought to contribute to muscle building and muscle cell and fiber enhancement. Studies show that consumption of milk after hard workouts resulted in more muscle growth compared to the same workouts followed by carbohydrates.

Cottage cheese is a concentrated source of protein with 28 grams in a one-cup, eight-ounce serving. Like other dairy sources, cottage cheese protein is high in the muscle-building amino acid, leucine. And as with milk and dairy, you may choose from fat-free, low-fat, or full-fat versions. As dairy fats tend to be high in saturated fats, you are encouraged to opt for the fat-free or low-fat versions.

Eggs provide quality protein with one egg containing six grams of protein, and only 70 calories. Eggs are high in the amino acid leucine, which is a key muscle-building component of protein. Eggs have additional nutritional benefits, including choline and B vitamins, and are recommended to be eaten despite containing cholesterol. If you prefer, increase your consumption of egg whites, which are cholesterol-free and almost pure protein.

Fish and Seafood Protein Sources

Salmon is a coldwater fish that is high in omega-3 fatty acids, which provide antioxidant benefits and are believed to contribute to muscle growth. There are 34 grams of protein in a six-ounce serving of lean salmon steak. Canned salmon is similarly high in protein and nutrients. Other coldwater fish like cod, sea bass, turbot, mackerel, and sardines are also recommended as is tuna, discussed next.

Tuna is even a bit higher in protein than salmon, with 40 grams in a six-ounce serving, plus vitamin A and B vitamins, including B6, B12, and niacin, all of which contribute to energy and workout performance. Tuna also has a high level of antioxidant omega-3 acids, which are believed to slow the rate of age-related muscle loss. As with salmon, canned tuna is similarly high in protein and nutrients, compared with fresh.

Shrimp is another high-protein seafood choice, with 36 grams of protein in a six-ounce serving. Shrimp are high in the muscle-building amino acid leucine. With minimal fats and virtually no carbohydrates, a six-ounce serving of shrimp contains only 144 calories.

Scallops are almost identical to shrimp in their nutritional composition but are a little higher in calories and protein with 40 grams in a six-ounce serving.

Meat Protein Sources

Chicken breast, served lean with skin removed and any visible fat cut away, is very high in protein with 26 grams of pure protein in a three-ounce serving or 52 grams in a six-ounce piece. There are also good amounts of vitamins B6 and niacin, which are credited with helping your body functioning during exercise and creating favorable conditions for muscle growth.

Lean beef is close to chicken breast in providing a high level of protein, but the challenge is to select beef that is truly low in fat. Avoid fatty cut by choosing a lean steak and cut away all visible fat. Avoid cuts that are marbled with fat that cannot be removed. When using ground beef, select the 95 percent lean option, which is far lower in saturated fat calories: a three-ounce serving of 95 percent lean beef contains 145 calories compared to 228 calories for 70 percent lean beef.

Turkey breast is very lean white meat, and when served without skin (which may contain a layer of fat), it provides 25 grams of protein in a three-ounce serving. The 100 calories in this serving are almost all fat and carbohydrate-free, and like chicken breast, high in muscle-building B vitamins, especially niacin.

Plant Sources of Protein

There are a few plant-based foods that contain a complete protein with the nine essential amino acids we need in our diets, but most plant sources are incomplete and need to be supplemented by other plant-based sources that are complementary:

➤ A combination of beans, legumes, and grains provide all necessary amino acids for nutritionally complete protein.

➤ For example, a meal made with black, pinto, or kidney beans, combined with brown rice or wheat-based pasta, provides nutritionally complete protein.

➤ However, protein levels in animal-derived foods are far more concentrated and provide more protein per ounce or measure compared to plant-sourced protein.,

Soybeans are probably the best-known plant source of complete protein with good reason. There are 14 grams of protein in ½-cup of cooked soybeans with beneficial unsaturated fats, vitamin K, and the important minerals, iron and phosphorus. You may also choose immature fresh or frozen soybeans, called **edamame**. One cup of edamame beans contains 17 grams of protein and eight grams of fiber, which aids digestion. It contains significant amounts of manganese and vitamin K, plus folate, which is credited with helping to process amino acids and optimize muscle growth among middle-aged and older people.

Quinoa is a grain that has complete, or nearly complete, protein, plus a large amount of unrefined, healthy carbohydrates for energy. One cup of cooked quinoa contains eight grams of protein, along with 40 grams of carbohydrates and five grams of digestion-supporting fiber. Its nutrients include phosphorus and magnesium, which aids the function of the nervous system's coordination with skeletal muscles.

Beans, including kidney, lima, black, and pinto, are a good source of vegetative-source protein with 15 grams of protein in one cup of cooked beans. As noted above, beans need to be paired with grains and cereals, like rice, oats, quinoa, wheat, and rye (in bread or pasta, for example). Beans are rich in nutrients, including B vitamins and the minerals iron, phosphorus, and magnesium.

Other nutritional plant sources of protein include brown rice, oats, chickpeas, peanuts, almonds, and buckwheat (used in baking instead of flour). Grains and cereals are lower than beans and legumes in protein and higher in carbohydrates. Nuts are higher than most foods in oils, which are unsaturated and beneficial, but high in calories, so be careful how many you eat.

Is There an Ideal Diet?

Walk into a bookstore and look for the section for books on diet. You will need time just to read the titles because the number of diets that are recommended is extensive. There are several reasons for this:

> Many people need help and guidance on weight loss and for managing conditions and illnesses: diabetes, heart disease, hypertension, cancers, immune disorders, and psychological problems among others.

> There is generally a belief that there is a magic diet, a silver bullet solution to lose weight, build muscle, cure disease, and live longer.

> Diet is all about eating, and people generally take eating very seriously as evidenced by the size of the cookbook section at the bookstore.

Let's take a quick look at some of the diets that are popular today, but with the understanding that while there are responsible ways to help with weight control and prevent or alleviate certain diseases, there is no single amazing diet that is the solution for everyone's problems. There is no "one size fits all" die because each of us has our own unique physiology, our own metabolic rate, our own sensitivities.

Popular Diets

Fasting has emerged recently as a way to health, happiness and a longer life, but you need to know that while the research involving worms and mice has been encouraging, the studies involving humans are mostly in the early stages. The more common approaches are intermittent fasting, conducted on a daily, repeating basis, such as the 16:8 fasting diet, which allows eating during an eight-hour period (e.g., 8 a.m. to 4 p.m.), and nothing to eat for the next 16 hours (4 p.m. to 8 a.m.). There are stricter versions, like 18:6. Alternatively, some try prolonged fasting, going for 24- or even 48- hour fasts, followed by a day of unlimited eating. People who practice this tend not to overeat on the non-fast days because their stomachs shrink a bit during the fast period,

> As a weightlifter seeking to build muscles, fasting diets are not advised for you.

Paleo diets harken back to paleolithic, simpler times when our distant ancestors were hunter-gatherers and ate "off the land," which means whatever they could find. This inspires diets today that avoid all refined and processed foods (which is commendable) and based on foods that our bodies evolved over millions of years to digest effectively.

According to the Mayo Clinic, a paleo diet usually includes vegetables, fruits, nuts and seeds, lean meats, and fish, which are the foods that could be gained by hunting and gathering. A paleo diet limits foods like dairy products, grains and legumes, and potatoes that became available when farming and agriculture started around 10,000 years ago. Added salt is also avoided. Overall, the paleo diet is acknowledged as healthy and wholesome as long as the ratios of macronutrients are respected, and a diversity of foods is included so that adequate amounts of vitamins and minerals are included.

Keto diet, short for ketogenic, has a very specific objective: rapid weight loss through stimulation of fat burning. This is achieved by following a very high-fat, very low-carbohydrate diet, essentially replacing the carbs with fats. This results in a metabolic condition called ketosis, which is highly efficient in using stored and dietary fat, instead of carbs and stored glycogen, for energy. You burn fat; you lose weight. Another quality is the conversion of fat stored in the liver to ketones, which supply energy to the brain. Also, the keto diet has been shown to lower blood sugar and insulin levels, which may contribute to the prevention or reduction of diabetes and other disorders. Other benefits are a feeling of fullness (satiety) that reduces cravings to eat or snack and improved mood. Studies of the longer-term effects of keto and other very low-carb diets are underway.

While the keto diet appears to be effective for weight loss, it may not include sufficient protein for building muscle mass; at least 30 percent of your diet should be protein.

Mediterranean diet. Let's conclude with a diet that is not only gaining broad acceptance, but it is the closest to the ideal diet everyone is searching for. It includes a wide range of wholesome and great-tasting foods, is affordable, is credited by the medical community as being heart-healthy, and may help slow the onset of many other diseases, from diabetes to cancer.

This diet is based on the practices of long-term residents of the Mediterranean Basin, including parts of Italy, Spain, and France, who tend to live healthier, longer lives. But importantly, these people practice a lifestyle that includes not only diet, but also being physically active all their lives, keeping their weight at normal levels, and having a positive attitude towards life.

The components of the Mediterranean diet:

➤ A variety of fresh vegetables, fresh and dried fruits, nuts, and seeds, whole grains and cereals, fish, lean meat in small servings (e.g., six ounces), moderate quantities of dairy (mostly as cheese), eggs, extra virgin olive oil, and wine, mostly red, consumed in moderation.

Whatever diet you choose, remember that as a weightlifter and builder of strength and muscle, you need sufficient protein in your diet, and you should select foods that are low in saturated fats. Avoid salty, processed foods, fried foods, and anything containing large amounts of sugar. The next section details the good and bad sources of foods.

Food Sources: Good and Bad

The types and sources of the three macronutrients have been discussed in detail, but to summarize, here is a quick checklist of the good and the bad. While this chapter has been devoted to helping you to understand the foods that are most beneficial to your health and to improve your level of physical fitness, build muscle and make you stronger, there are sources of carbohydrates, proteins, and fat that you should avoid. To help your dietary planning, we've listed both the recommended sources of your macronutrients and the foods that have been designated as undesirable and potentially harmful.

According to nutritionists at MD Anderson Cancer Center:

Recommended carbohydrates sources include:

➤ Dairy products, including milk, yogurt, and cottage cheese, but with a preference for low-fat or non-fat since full-fat dairy products are high in saturated fats and calories. Non-dairy substitutes made from soy, almonds, and oats are also good sources of carbs. Dairy products also provide high-quality complete protein.

➤ Vegetables, which can be eaten without limitation since they are low in calories and rich in vitamins and minerals. Select a variety of colors (green, yellow, red, purple) which will provide a diversity of micronutrients.

➤ Fruits are high in natural sugars (which is why they taste sweet) and micronutrients. Fruit should be eaten without added sugar and in natural, solid form to preserve pulp, which adds valuable fiber. Many juices have added sugar and the pulp has been removed.

➤ Beans, peas, and lentils, known as legumes, provide high levels of carbohydrates, plus fiber and many of the 20 amino acids that comprise protein.

➤ Whole grains, including whole wheat, rye, buckwheat, spelt, corn, and oats, are high in carbs and are excellent sources of vitamin B and fiber. Refined grains do not have these added qualities.

Carbohydrate sources to avoid:

➤ Refined flours and sugar, found in crackers, most breads, cookies, breakfast cereals, and sugar, in most fruit juices, soft drinks, most athletic performance beverages, and candy.

Recommended protein sources include:

➤ Beans, including black, pinto, and kidney beans, plus lentils and soy products. Except for soy, the proteins are incomplete and need supplementation with grains and cereals.

➤ Nuts and seeds, including nut butters (sugar-free versions).

➤ Whole grains, including quinoa, rye, wheat, spelt, corn, and soy, with the caveat that the amino acids do not comprise complete protein.

➤ Animal protein from meat, poultry, fish and seafood, dairy, and eggs.

Protein sources to avoid:

➤ Processed meats, like sausages, salami, bacon, frankfurters (hot dogs), and canned lunch meats.

➤ Consumption of lean red meats should be limited to 18 ounces per week.

Recommended fat sources include:

➤ Vegetable oils, especially extra virgin olive oil, avocado oil, and canola oil, and secondarily, oils from corn, sunflower, and safflower.

➤ Fatty fish, notably coldwater salmon, tuna, mackerel, and sardines.

➢ Flax seeds, chia seeds, avocados, and olives.

➢ Nuts and seeds, and again, natural nut butters, no sugar added.

Fat sources to avoid:

➢ Fried foods, which are made with refined flour and absorb large amounts of oils that contain trans fats.

➢ Animal sources, including full-fat dairy like milk, butter, yogurt, cream cheese, and the fats on meats and poultry.

➢ Vegetable oils from coconut and palm sources, shortening (used in baking), soft tub margarines, and most packaged baked goods (read the labels for fat content).

Now, on to Chapter 7 and dismissing some common misconceptions about working out, getting into shape, building muscles, and gaining strength when you are 40-plus.

Chapter 7:

Common Misconceptions About Fitness After 40

What to believe? You are middle-aged and about to begin a serious strengthening and fitness program. Is it safe? Should you be doing this at your age? Maybe you've been warned by others or have concerns of your own. Let's get to the facts.

1. You're too old to be lifting weights and doing cardio workouts.

Let's put this myth to bed quickly. There is no age limit to becoming fit. If you are male or female, age 40, 50, or 60, you actually need a good exercise program more now than when you were younger. Yes, it would have been easier when you had the muscles and arteries of a 20-year-old, but in those days, your body took care of itself. Now your metabolism is slower, the fat tends to accumulate more easily, and you are losing muscle mass. Your bones may be getting more porous and susceptible to breakage. A good resistance and aerobics program can reverse those symptoms of aging. If you're new to this and out of shape, see your doctor first, as we advise in Chapter 4, get the proper cautions, then get to work bringing your body back to its fitness and health potential.

2. You need to spend more time working out.

Being middle-age is not a rationale for extending your workouts. Less is more when you perform an intense, quality workout, so there's no basis for overdoing it or wasting time you may need elsewhere. Even when time precludes a full workout at the health club, you can still spend 20 minutes at home giving yourself a good workout with weights or by doing bodyweight calisthenics. Even when there's no time pressure, a complete weightlifting or cardiovascular workout can be done in 40 minutes or less. Any more than that may lead to overwork injuries, especially in middle age, so control your time to optimize the workout.

3. You should not do high-intensity workouts.

It all depends what is meant by intensity. For weightlifting, there is overwhelming evidence that you can build muscle in middle-age as long as you work up to your peak levels gradually and find the sweet spot between too little weight and too much. Here's a reminder of the recommendations in the book. After warming up, perform between eight and 10 reps with weights you can just make to those last one or two reps. If you can't do more than less than eight, it's too heavy, and if you can do more than 10, the weight is too light. Do three sets of eight to 10 reps with the optimal weight and your workout will have all the intensity you need.

4. You do not have time to workout.

Maybe you are at a point in your career when it's all on the line, and you need to get to work early and stay late. You feel that 30 or 40 minutes out of your day just isn't affordable to you. Recalling Parkinson's law that work expands to fill the available time, you should re-evaluate your work ethic; you may realize that you do have more discretionary time. Ask yourself if you really don't have the time or is it that you don't have the motivation to exercise, get stronger, and be fit? If you've jumped to this chapter before reading the book, head back to Chapter 5 and read about motivation and commitment. You also have the option to break up your workouts to a few minutes here and there throughout the day, getting up and moving around. Studies confirm that you can burn the calories, challenge the muscles, and strengthen the heart in short bursts.

5. Running is dangerous and should be avoided.

Running at middle-age does have some risks. especially for your joints, and connective tissues, so we need to find the ideal, safe way to run. Ideally, you can run on a treadmill, which cushions your steps, and is far less likely to bother your knees, which are the most susceptible to wear and tear as the years go by. If you do want to run outdoors, try for softer surfaces like grass or trails through forests and parks. Wear a good pair of running shoes to cushion and also prevent your foot from pronating, or rolling. If running becomes painful, consider switching to race walking, which doesn't pound the joints, yet can give you a good cardio workout.

6. Either diet or exercise will keep weight down, you don't need both.

This is covered in Chapter 6, but to hit the key points: diet is by far the more influential in managing your weight. Calories in, calories out (how many calories you digest vs. how many you burn) is the prevailing scientific principle, and it is far easier to resist ingesting the 500-calorie pair of iced doughnuts or a cup of full-fat ice cream than to have to run or walk five miles to burn those calories off. Especially since studies prove that calories burned through exercise are partially offset by a slower metabolism when you're resting or asleep. The best way to lose weight is to follow a responsible diet (not a fad diet) and eat less while you continue your fitness program. Increase the protein in your diet to better build muscles, keep you fuller longer, and less likely to snack.

7. **It's too late to lose belly fat.**

The same "calories in, calories out" principle applies here as well. If you burn more calories in a given period than you consume and digest, your weight will go down, and excess fat will be what is lost. Now, it's true that fat tends to accumulate around your gut as you get older and your metabolism slows down. But even that fat can't stay for long if you maintain a good caloric deficit. Unfortunately, we can't "spot reduce" fat, meaning abdominal exercises like leg raises and planks, will harden the muscles but will have no direct effect on the belly fat. If you want to lose fat, the best approach is to lose weight through a combination of diet and exercise.

Conclusion

This book was written for anyone who is over age 40 and is thinking that it's time to get into good physical shape, either for the first time or to return to the good condition of when you were younger. If you are concerned that it may be too late for you, that you've waited too long to begin or to resume working out, this book assures you that it's not too late, In fact, your timing is excellent.

Let's recap by reviewing the key points of what the book has covered.

Your body has evolved. It is no longer the body of when you were 20 or even 30; your metabolism is slowing, imperceptibly but gradually, year after year, and you have been losing muscle mass, and gaining fat. These changes may be obvious, or subtle, but they are happening as a natural part of the aging process. But these changes are not inevitable and can be slowed, stopped, or even reversed by a well-planned fitness program involving weightlifting and other resistance exercises, cardiovascular conditioning, and a responsible diet.

Stronger after 40? Can you really build muscles and get stronger after 40? Yes, because there is science behind the workouts, the sweat, and exertion. It's called hypertrophy, the process of tearing down muscle cells and fiber while lifting weights, and then resting while your body repairs the damage by adding protein and overbuilds slightly. Over time, the overbuilding accumulates, creating larger, stronger muscles. This process may happen more slowly at age 40 or 50, but it happens nonetheless.

➤ You can exercise hard, just not the same old way.

➤ Your age is not a barrier to achieving serious muscle bulk and definition once you learn how to perform the right exercises with the right weights and routines.

Lifting heavy weights. The question of how much weight to lift safely, yet effectively, leads to options from many reps of light weights to very few — one, two, or three — reps that you can barely handle. The optimal weights are those you can lift eight to 10 times with the last rep being really tough to lift, pull, or push all the way. So, yes, you can lift heavy weights as long as you follow the eight-to-10 reps maximum.

Motivation, commitment, consistency. A successful muscle-building, strength, and fitness program requires the motivation to begin, but even more importantly, you need an unshakeable commitment to consistently renew your dedication to weightlifting and cardiovascular training over the long term:

➤ Without motivation, getting started might be put off indefinitely, or you may start your workouts half-heartedly. But motivation is only the stimulus, the catalyst to get you started; it's *commitment and consistency* that will drive you to achieve your muscle-building and fitness goals. Without commitment and consistency in your progressive training, you may be tempted to quit or slow down, and that will not get you where you need to go.

➤ Begin every day with a self-image of who you want to be. Picture those bigger biceps, the well-defined chest and abdominals, the powerful legs, the flat gut. Resolve every morning, as soon as you wake up, to achieve that body, that strength, vitality, and energy.

➤ Consistency requires willpower, and you know you have it deep within. You can call on it to pull on those gym shorts and workout shoes every day and give your muscles and your heart the conditioning they need and deserve as you renew your effort and commitment to longevity and health.

➤ Consider each workout to be an investment in long-term physical equity. Like building a solid wall, a few bricks and mortar at a time, hypertrophy slowly but consistently increases muscle tissue. Commit to long-term growth.

➤ Progress may be slow at middle-age, imperceptible on a daily or weekly basis, but by making your workouts a continuing routine over the months and years, your commitment to consistency will pay off with the body you dream of. Slow progress is better than no progress, and with tenacity and patience, great results will be there for you.

➤ Your workouts will vary in their intensity, and some days will feel fulfilling and other days less so. But there are no bad workouts — showing up is what it takes — because the only "bad" workout is the one you didn't do. Remember the tip: on days when it's tough to even think about working out, tell yourself you'll just take it easy with a few dumbbell lifts, a few push-ups, but know that once you get started and warmed up, your energy will return and you'll put in a good workout.

You can do this. This book has you covered with ways to get started and maintain your commitment and resolve to reach your muscle, strength, and fitness objectives. You have seen the workouts of celebrity athletes, from James Bond to The Rock, and while you are not going to follow their extreme workouts, you can be inspired by their examples of dedication and discipline.

Do no harm. In presenting a range of weightlifting exercises and calisthenics, you have noted the upfront warning of do no harm and be respectful of your age and your body. Warm up and start slowly with weights more on the lighter side until you get the hang of it.

Where to workout? You may have access to a well-equipped health club, fitness center, or gym and will be able to use free weights, exercise machines with cables to pull and handles to push, plus rubber stretch bands (which can replicate many weight and machine movements), and treadmill and elliptical machines for cardiovascular workouts. Or you may want a home gym with some free weights, like dumbbells and barbells, rubber stretch bands and tubes, and a bar for pull-ups and chin-ups.

Another good option, which requires almost no equipment, is bodyweight calisthenics, which you can perform at home or anywhere. Your bodyweight actually can provide quite a lot of resistance; think of how much weight you are lifting when you do push-ups, squats, or pull-ups.

Full-body workout. The seven weightlifting and seven calisthenics exercises are more than enough for you to achieve full-body workouts challenging every muscle group. You are encouraged to draw your routines from both groups if you have the weights; otherwise, you can achieve equally impressive results entirely with bodyweight calisthenics. Each exercise includes a link to a video demonstration with good instructions from professional trainers so you can learn and perform the movements safely and effectively.

Rest and recovery. You have been instructed in the importance of rest and recovery since the process of hypertrophy takes time, and even more as you get older. Muscle groups should have at least one day of rest, preferable two, between resistance workouts. You have the choice of working the full body and resting for two or three days, or working out more frequently and limiting each workout to one or two muscle groups, like arms and shoulders on Monday, chest and core on Tuesday, legs on Wednesday, and back to arms and shoulders on Thursday. You have the freedom to select the routines and timing that work for you. You should aim to work each muscle group at least two times each week.

Metabolic rate. You've received a briefing on your metabolism to understand what it is, how it affects your bodily functions, and why and how it slows as the years pass. The importance of being highly motivated to start your strengthening and fitness program is again emphasized as is the need for the commitment to keep your fitness program going over the long term, making it a valued component of your lifestyle. Hopefully, the inspirational quotes in that section will give you added drive.

You are what you eat. The subject of diet was covered in detail and sought to bring clarity to the often misunderstood role of carbohydrates, proteins, and fats — the macronutrients — in giving our bodies energy, structure, and function. CICO, the principle of calories in, calories out, makes it evident that there is no way to avoid taking in fewer calories than you burn each day if you want to lose weight.

➤ The extra importance of **protein** for weightlifters and exercise enthusiasts in middle age is explained, and there is a list of recommended sources of healthy protein from both animal and plant sources.

➤ Different popular diets were covered, and you are encouraged to follow a diet like the Mediterranean, which encourages a wide assortment of fruit and vegetables, lean meat and fish, grains, beans and cereals, nuts and seeds, olive oil, and even red wine, in moderation.

➤ Those who follow this diet eat for pleasure as well as for health and fitness and maintain a physically active lifestyle.

Misconceptions about fitness. We concluded with some of the popular misconceptions about weightlifting and exercising at age 40-plus and provided reassurance that *yes, you can,* and *yes, you should* stay healthier, stronger, less likely to suffer injuries, and help resist diseases. You actually do have the time to exercise, despite a busy schedule, you can, and should, lift heavy weights. Both diet and exercise are needed for maintaining a healthy weight, and yes, you can burn fat at your age.

Let's go. If you have not yet started your strengthening and fitness program, what are you waiting for? I would sum up by telling you:

➤ "The best time to start was yesterday. The second-best time is now."

I am CJD Fitness founder Baz Thompson, a CYQ Master Personal Trainer who has helped hundreds of people like you achieve their fitness goals. I work with professional athletes as well as coaching global executives and people of all ages. and I have enjoyed this opportunity to be working with you.

In closing, I would like to ask that if you have benefitted from reading this book, and believe that others who have reached or surpassed age 40 and want to get into shape could benefit as well, please consider giving this book a favorable review on Amazon. This will send a signal to other potential readers who need help and will reassure them that this book is for them.

I trust you will experience excellent health and well-being on the long road of life that lies before you and wish you my very best. Thank you for letting me share my knowledge with you.

Baz Thompson

Reference List

Alexander, H. (2020, June). What are macronutrients? *MD Anderson Cancer Center*. https://www.mdanderson.org/publications/focused-on-health/what-are-macronutrients-.h15-1593780.html

Barrell, A. (2020, Dec. 3). Should you workout when you're sore? *Medical News Today*. https://www.medicalnewstoday.com/articles/326892?utm_source=Sailthru%20Email&utm_medium=Email&utm_campaign=MNT%20Daily%20News&utm_content=2020-12-18&utm_country=&utm_hcp=&apid=25264436&utm_term=B

Brown, R. (2016, Sept. 16). Top 5 fitness myths of adults over 50. *Next Avenue*. https://www.nextavenue.org/top-5-fitness-myths-among-adults-over-50/

Cassetty, S. (2020, Sept. 11). The CICO diet: how it does and does not work for weight loss. *Today*. https://www.today.com/health/what-cico-diet-all-about-calories-calories-out-diet-t191457

Cathe. (2019, April 11). What impact does exercise have on blood lipids? https://cathe.com/what-impact-does-exercise-have-on-blood-lipids/

Current Biology. (2016). Constrained total energy expenditure and metabolic adaptation to physical activity in adult humans. https://www.cell.com/current-biology/fulltext/S0960-9822(15)01577-8

da Silva, J., Vinagre, C. et al. (2011, Sept. 9). Resistance training changes LDL metabolism in normolipidemic subjects: a study with a nanoemulsion mimetic of LDL. *Atherosclerosis*. https://www.atherosclerosis-journal.com/article/S0021-9150(11)00818-5/abstract

Davis, N. (2019, March 25). Try this: 17 exercises to relieve upper back pain, neck pain, and more. *Healthline*. https://www.healthline.com/health/fitness-exercise/upper-back-pain-exercises?slot_pos=article_2&utm_source=Sailthru%20Email&utm_medium=Email&utm_campaign=generalhealth&utm_content=2020-12-01&apid=25264436&rvid=0fcaeb66b8efed5fc78f73c81adf7036378bf5e4be033e89cfcfa2700293b230

Eliza. (2019, Sept. 16). 5 fitness over 40 myths debunked. *Eliza Tips*.
https://elizadoalot.com/5-fitness-over-40-myths-debunked/

Frontera, W., Hughes, V., et al. (2000, April). Aging of skeletal muscle: a 12-yr longitudinal study. *Journal of Applied Physiology*. https://pubmed.ncbi.nlm.nih.gov/10749826/

Gunnars, K. (2019, March 8). 10 science-backed reasons to eat more protein. *Healthline*.
https://www.healthline.com/nutrition/10-reasons-to-eat-more-protein

Harvard Health Publishing. (2016, February). Preserve your muscle mass.
https://www.health.harvard.edu/staying-healthy/preserve-your-muscle-mass/

Ho, S., Dhaliwal, S., et al. (2012, Aug. 28). The effect of 12 weeks of aerobic, resistance or combination exercise training on cardiovascular risk factors in the overweight and obese in a randomized trial. *BMC Public Health*.
https://www.ncbi.nlm.nih.gov/pmc/articles/PMC3487794/

Karen. (2019, Sept. 27). Get fit over 40 by rejecting 5 fitness myths. *Well Balanced Women*.
https://wellbalancedwomen.com/5-fitness-myths-women-over-40/

Mayo Clinic Staff. (2020). Exercise: a drug-free approach to lowering high blood pressure.
https://www.mayoclinic.org/diseases-conditions/high-blood-pressure/in-depth/high-blood-pressure/art-20045206

Mayo Clinic Staff. (2020). Exercise and chronic disease: get the facts.
https://www.mayoclinic.org/healthy-lifestyle/fitness/in-depth/exercise-and-chronic-disease/art-20046049

Mayo Clinic Staff. (2020). Nutrition and healthy eating. Paleo diet: what is it and why is it so popular? https://www.mayoclinic.org/healthy-lifestyle/nutrition-and-healthy-eating/in-depth/paleo-diet/art-20111182

National Heart, Lung, and Blood Institute. (2020). Calculate your body mass index.
https://www.nhlbi.nih.gov/health/educational/lose_wt/BMI/bmicalc.htm

National Osteoporosis Foundation. (2020). Osteoporosis exercises for strong bones.
https://www.nof.org/patients/treatment/exercisesafe-movement/osteoporosis-exercise-for-strong-bones/

Raman, R. (2017, Sept. 24). Why your metabolism slows down with age. *Healthline*.
https://www.healthline.com/nutrition/metabolism-and-age

Siddique, H. (2016, Jan. 28). Exercise alone won't cause weight loss, study shows. *The Guardian*. https://www.theguardian.com/science/2016/jan/28/study-reveals-that-exercise-alone-wont-cause-weight-loss

Story, C. (2019, Jan. 9). Lowering your high cholesterol: 6 exercises that will pay off. *Healthline*. https://www.healthline.com/health/high-cholesterol/treating-with-statins/best-exercises

Tinsley, G. (2018, Jan. 21). 26 foods that help you build lean muscle. *Healthline*. https://www.healthline.com/nutrition/26-muscle-building-foods

Tzankoff, S., Norris, A. (1977, Dec. 1). Effects of muscle mass decrease on age-related BMR changes. *Journal of Applied Physiology*. https://journals.physiology.org/doi/pdf/10.1152/jappl.1977.43.6.1001

U.S. News & World Report. (2021). Keto diet. https://health.usnews.com/best-diet/keto-diet

Van Pelt, R., Pones, P., et al. (1997, October). Regular exercise and the age-related decline in resting metabolic rate in women. *Journal of Clinical Endocrinol Metabolism*. https://pubmed.ncbi.nlm.nih.gov/9329340/

WebMD. (2020). 6 Exercises to help your knees. https://www.webmd.com/pain-management/knee-pain/injury-knee-pain-16/slideshow-knee-exercises?ecd=wnl_spr_122020&ctr=wnl-spr-122020_nsl-Bodymodule_Position3&mb=MukfT6opS3AxbF5kSEwI0ng0WleHxvIqssh%40W3619r4%3d

Reference List for Images

Fig 1. Herman, Scott. (2010, March 27). How to: dumbbell incline chest press. YouTube. https://www.youtube.com/watch?v=8iPEnn-ltC8

Fig 2. Herman, Scott. (2010, April 10). How to: seated low row. YouTube. https://www.youtube.com/watch?v=GZbfZ033f74

Fig 3. IntoSport. (2019, Dec. 8). Dumbbell split squat - fitness gym training. YouTube. https://www.youtube.com/watch?v=MEG6blZtUpc

Fig 4. Herman, Scott. (2012, Dec. 29). How to: dumbbell bent-over row. YouTube. https://www.youtube.com/watch?v=6TSP1TRMUzs

Fig 5. Calabrese, A. (2014, Sept. 1). How to upright row - proper form and tips. YouTube. https://www.youtube.com/watch?v=VIoihl5ZZzM

Fig 6. Azar, B. (2012, Aug. 21). How to do a barbell curl/arm workout. Howcast/YouTube. https://www.youtube.com/watch?v=kwG2ipFRgfo

Fig 7. Herman, S. (2010, Fe. 1). How to: dumbbell lateral side raise. YouTube. https://www.youtube.com/watch?v=3VcKaXpzqRo

Fig 8. Henson, J. (2015, June 18). How to do a proper plank. Body Mind Wellness Clinic/YouTube. https://www.youtube.com/watch?v=gvHVdNVBu6s

Fig 9. McKee, K. (2015, Dec. 11). How to do a body-weight squat. Health Magazine/YouTube. https://www.youtube.com/watch?v=LyidZ42Iy9Q

Fig 10. Syuki, R. (2020, May 30). How to do lying leg raises for abs. YouTube. https://www.youtube.com/watch?v=UvcTNVbjTYo

Fig 11. Rilinger, H. (2015, Aug. 25). How to do a push-up. Dr. Oz/YouTube. https://www.youtube.com/watch?v=rjc0O7OXS3g

Fig 12. Crossfit. (2019, Feb. 1). The strict pull-up. YouTube. https://www.youtube.com/watch?v=HRV5YKKaeVw

Fig 13. Critical Bench. (2018, Sep. 24). Hanging leg raise done right. YouTube. https://www.youtube.com/watch?v=lS5B0MmLgZs

Fig 14. Herman, S. (2011, Oct. 1). How to: bench dips. YouTube. Fig https://www.youtube.com/watch?v=c3ZGl4pAwZ4

Printed in Great Britain
by Amazon

56882115R00066